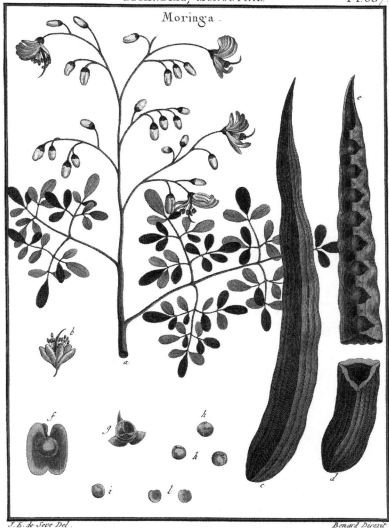

Moringa.

J. E. de Seve Del.　　Benard Direxit

HISTOIRE NATURELLE, *Botanique*.

Reproduced from "Encyclopedie Méthodique" by Lamarck
Published by Panckouke, 1801

MIRACLE TREE

MIRACLE TREE

by
Monica G. Marcu, PHARM. D., PH. D.

Published by:

sound**concepts**

782 S. Automall Drive, Suite A
American Fork, UT 84003
soundconcepts.com

The information in this book is for educational purposes only and should not be used to diagnose and treat diseases. All serious health conditions should be treated by a competent health practitioner. Neither the publisher nor the author of this book in any way dispense medical advice, prescribe remedies, or assume responsibility for those who choose to treat themselves.

ISBN 1-49594-609-6
Printed in the United States of America

Dedicated to all the people who study,
promote or use Moringa...
Dedicated to all my beloved trees.

"The wonder is that we can see these trees and not wonder more."

Ralph Waldo Emerson

Table of Contents

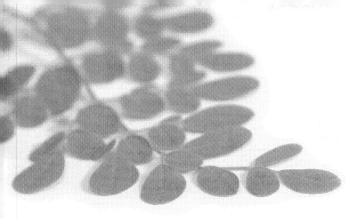

PREFACE

I have always been enchanted by trees. I looked at them, studied them, and climbed them. I hugged them shamelessly, I envied those trees. I talked to them often; and photographed them thousands of times. Some of my photographs have names such as: "The Never Enough Trees" and, indeed, the trees were never enough to me. Admittedly, this might sound rather eccentric, especially when you know I am, after all, a "cold-blooded" scientist. The extraordinary thing in this whole story is one good day, life suddenly prompted me to write a book about…a tree, or, to be more precise, an extraordinary tree. Well, this surprise found me ripe. I believe my whole life I was unknowingly preparing myself to write This Book. But maybe I should not call it a "surprise", rather an expected order of things: there must have been so much love for trees, so much passion for Nature within my heart, that life compelled me to express myself in this project.

It is my hope that I will be able to match life's expectations and bring you the unbelievable, beautiful story of one of our greatest trees, Moringa. A tree rich in the most precious nutrients that has wisely chosen to grow where it is most needed – in arid, drought-plagued areas of our world. Moringa, a resilient tree, inherently resistant to many diseases, can also help our body heal itself from some of its diseases. It's a tree that can amazingly grow 5-6 meters (yards) in a year, despite minimum rainfall. Moringa is a tree that brings hope to malnourished children while drying the tears of their mothers. No wonder it is surrounded by legends and praise, awe and respect. Moringa bears a variety of suggestive names around the world such as: "Miracle Tree", "Mother's Best Friend", and "Never Die". It has been more than overwhelming to learn about the many uses of Moringa, and, during this process, I came to love and talk about her as a close friend. Don't be surprised to notice my affection here and there, while reading this short book about a great being.

After a comprehensive introduction, this book is organized in chapters explaining the main beneficial nutrients and compounds found in Moringa. The subsequent chapters show how Moringa can improve our general health. My wish is that anybody who reads this book may understand the extraordinary value of this plant for humanity. The mission was difficult; Moringa has hundreds of substances such as vitamins, enzymes, amino acids, fats, minerals, specific phytochemicals (plant-derived), each with clear importance and numerous applications in healing and nutrition. I tried to remain objective and impartial, although it is hard not to be excited and fascinated by Moringa. In comparable amounts (gram per gram), Moringa contains more vitamin C than oranges, three times the iron of spinach, and four times the calcium found in milk. Combine these with significant amounts of proteins and oils, a great taste, and the presence of beneficial antioxidant (antiaging) and anti-inflamma-tory substances and you will come to understand why they call her a Miracle Tree.

*Keep a green tree in your heart
and perhaps a singing bird will come.*

Chinese Proverb

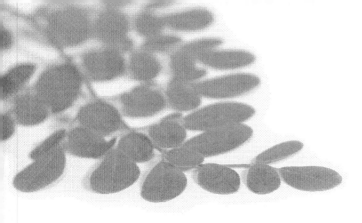

INTRODUCING MORINGA

Identity and Appearance

I would like to warmly introduce to you *Moringa oleifera,* a plant of the family called Moringaceae. Actually, *Moringa oleifera* is the most studied of 14 species of Moringa trees. It is commonly known as the "drumstick tree", "horseradish tree" (the root tastes similar to horseradish) or "radish tree", but has hundreds of other names around the world. I will call it Moringa.

Moringa is a small, fast-growing shrub or tree that can reach 12 m (36 ft.) in height at maturity and can live for up to 20 years. A short but intense life...a life in the fast lane: Moringa is perhaps the fastest-grow-ing of all trees as it can reach 3 m (9 ft.) in just 10 months after the seed is planted. She has deep roots, and therefore she can survive in dry regions, and a wide-open crown with a single stem.

Moringa is a compassionate tree: an ideal tree for agro-forestry, her branches can be easily trimmed to regulate shade, and her open crown allows the sunlight to reach the garden vegetables below. Her wood is soft and the bark is light. Of all the Moringa tree's parts, the bark is the only part that can be toxic for human consumption.

I consider Moringa a very beautiful plant, especially the leaves. They are of a rare shape, deep green at maturity. The flowers are cream-colored, sweet-smelling, and are great for teas or as a honey source. The pods are triangular, rather long and legume-like in appearance. The seed husks are black and winged with a white inner seed. Around the world, Moringa is well-known for her many attributes and uses, wide adaptability and ease of growth. Most of her parts (leaves, pods, and flowers) are packed with exceptionally valuable nutrients for humans and animals.

Home Address

Moringa has her origin in Arabia and India (South of the Himalayan Mountains) but today she is common all over the tropics, from South Asia to West Africa. She is found in parts of East and South Africa, in many Pacific islands (from Kiribati to the Northern Marianas), in South and Central America and...everywhere indoors. Moringa does best where the temperature ranges from 25 to 40 degrees C

(77 to 104 degrees F) and annual rainfall is at least 500 mm. She grows well from sea level to 1,000 m (3,000 ft.) elevation. Historically, there is evidence that cultivation of Moringa in India dates back thousands of years, and the traditional Ayurvedic medicine used this tree to heal or prevent hundreds of diseases! The Greek, Roman and Egyptian people used parts of the plant for food and cosmetics. It is likely that Moringa was welcome everywhere.

Profession and Qualities

Moringa is a healer, food magician, beauty and beautician, a plant with surprising water purification capabilities, a best friend and humanitarian who works for so little. She is one of the most useful trees on earth, especially in semi-arid and drought-prone areas where she is often grown in courtyard gardens. Her succulent, protein-rich leaves are harvested daily for soups or salads. The amazing thing about the leaves is that they grow during the dry season and in times of drought, precisely when most other food growth is limited! The leaves and seeds (pods) are high in vitamins A, C, and B1, beneficial oils (similar to olive oil), and micronutrients. Where local diets lack these essential nutrients, Moringa makes a major contribution to human and animal health; in many cases, it can mean the difference between life and death. Absolutely no negative effects to daily consumption of Moringa leaves and seeds have ever been reported.

Moringa seeds contain about 35% oil that can be used for cooking, cosmetics (creams, soaps) and even lubricants. Since it does not turn rancid, it is excellent in salads, and burns without smoke. The oil can easily absorb volatile, scented substances; therefore, it is also used to manufacture perfumes. The seeds are often used to purify dirty, bacteria-laced water in places where there is nothing else that can be used as such. They are pounded into small pieces, wrapped in a cloth and placed into water containers. These miraculous seeds act as a flocculent, removing impurities and suspended bacteria, and other harmful organisms or particles out of the solution, leaving drinkable water above. From this perspective, Moringa seeds are considered to be better than the commonly used water purifier, aluminum sulfate, which is slightly toxic. Moringa is readily available where it is needed most, in regions where clean water is a permanent concern. Moringa represents an economical, viable solution to water purification. Remember, lack of drinkable water is one of the world's most serious health threats! Water-related diseases account for more than 80% of the world's sicknesses.

As a healing plant, Moringa is even more amazing. There is much evidence from around the world, from various traditions and cultures that have used this "Miracle Tree" for so many ailments and troubles. To mention just a few:

- The leaves are believed to have a stabilizing effect on blood pressure and control glucose levels. They are also used to treat anxiety, diarrhea and inflammation of the colon, skin infections, scurvy, intestinal parasites, and many other conditions.

- The seeds are used against fevers and tumors, while the seed oil is applied externally to relieve pain and swelling from gout or rheumatism. It is used internally for prostate and bladder ailments. The oil is considered an excellent tonic - no wonder, as it contains a multitude of vitamins and beneficial substances, as we shall further discuss.

It all might sound too good to be true, but many of the above traditional remedies have been supported by recent laboratory studies despite the fact that interest in Moringa's treasures only began a short time ago. The secret(s) might be in the multitude of nutrients, antioxidants, anti-inflammatory and antiaging compounds present in various parts of this tree. All together, they provide missing nutrients and balance the health, fight parasites and infections, support the natural immunity and fortify the body against stress and environmental harms. The "Never Die" tree does deserve her glory!

Moringa's benefits do not end here. This plant can be used as a domestic cleaning agent, dye (the wood yields a blue color), natural fertilizer (green manure), for rope-making or fencing around the garden.

In the following chapters, the amazing healing and nutritive properties of Moringa will be further explored and detailed. What proves to be the food and medicine of many people from less fortunate lands deserves attention and respect everywhere in the world. While many in the Western countries seem to benefit from too much food, or rather too many calories, which makes them overweight, they are actually undernourished since their diets are deficient in vital nutrients and antiaging (specifically plant-derived) substances. Moringa could be the low-caloric, low-salt, nutritious and concentrated solution. With a great taste!

"Now there are more overweight people in America than average-weight people. So overweight people are now average. Which means you've met your New Year's resolution."

Jay Leno

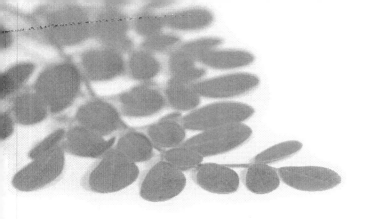

MORINGA IN THE NEWS

Moringa is famous and beloved in many parts of the world, while her fame is spreading and igniting exciting research projects in agriculture, forestry, botany, food and drug industries, health and cosmetics. Churches and charities, peace corps, and other humanitarian organizations such as Educational Concerns for Hunger Organization, or ECHO, Trees for Life - based in Wichita, Kansas - an organization that plants food-bearing trees in developing countries are interested in Moringa for obvious reasons. Church World Service (the U.S. National Council of Churches' global service and witness ministry) has recently organized the first-ever international conference on the Moringa tree, as an indigenous resource for fighting hunger and malnutrition. Participants from 27 countries, including 12 African nations, representatives from private industry, ministry officials, researchers, secular and

9

ecumenical non-governmental organizations were counted among the attendees.

The International Eye Foundation (based in Maryland, USA) is promoting Moringa for the prevention of childhood blindness (due to malnutrition) in poor countries. Indeed, Moringa, through her richness in vitamins, saves precious eyesight in the most vulnerable victims, children with vitamin A deficiency.

Newspapers and scientific journals mention Moringa more and more often. Until recently, this tree wasn't really known in the West, except to botanists. Today, Moringa - the very plant that desperate mothers from tropical countries use to save their malnourished children, is also featured as the exciting ingredient of a fancy skin rejuvenating cream. Researchers from Austria to Australia, Nicaragua and India, study Moringa's properties and growth. The National Science Foundation and National Geographic Society, together with other organizations, have started to finance the gathering of a collection of all Moringa species to gather more information about her many healthful properties.

Maybe among all the good news, the most moving stories came from the Senegalese project "Mother and Child Health." In an effort to combat child death and disease due to malnourishment, the use of locally-grown Moringa was proposed to infants, their nursing mothers and pregnant women.

Although Moringa grows in Africa, her leaves were rarely used as food before. In the classical approach to treat malnourished children, expensive industrial products such as whole milk powder, vegetable oil, or sugar were proposed. Most people could not afford them, but Moringa was local and easily grown. The medical staff advised parents to put a little bit of leaf powder in the child's food every day. Children were weighed before and after 2-3 months of such a supplement. (Many survived ONLY on Moringa leaves or seed powder!) Pictures were taken to document the results. When the women brought back their children a few months later, they were hardly recognizable! Malnourished mothers who did not produce enough milk for their babies, also recovered beyond all expectations on a Moringa diet. No wonder every villager started to grow Moringa around their houses, villages, and hospitals. And they spread the word.

It is difficult to find another comparable plant with such flexibility and richness. Corn, another example of an extraordinarily beneficial plant, has a multitude of uses, as well (for oil, cereal, sugar, alcohol, flour, animal fodder, and others), but it does not grow as fast or in poor weather conditions, and it is not known to contain such a wide gamut of vitamins, nutrients or medicinal compounds as Moringa.

Are you impressed? You should be.

...We respect and honor and admire you, O trees, for you represent both Peace and Power -though you are mighty you hurt no creature. Though you sustain us with your breath, you will give up your life to house and warm and teach us. We give thanks for your blessing upon our lives and upon our lands. May you fare well in this chosen place.

Druid Ceremony for Planting a Grove

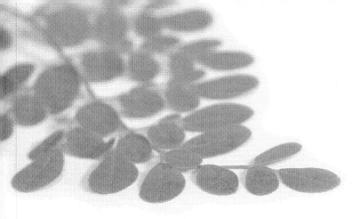

MORINGA,
THE MEDICAL·PLANT

As briefly mentioned when introducing Moringa, the plant is being used around the world by many cultures for a variety of ailments. It is time now to explore and explain in more detail some of the known and lesser known facts about her medicinal properties, active compounds, and their effects on humans and animals. Let me start with a short introduction on medicinal plants and their importance in human health.

Herbal (plant) medicine is the most ancient form of healthcare known to humankind. Plants as medicines are mentioned in historic documents dating back many thousands of years. Furthermore, many cultures, like Amazonian Indian tribes, with no written languages, depended on oral communication to convey information and traditions which were also rich in plant stories. Since

13

prehistoric times and continuing to our modern days, people from all over the world have grown or collected plants for the prevention and treatment of diseases. *Moringa oleifera* is one of the best examples. People have long known that botanical medicine provided a complete, safe system of healing and prevention of diseases.

The World Health Organization (WHO) estimates that nearly 80% of the world population is dependent on traditional medicine for primary healthcare. This is due to the fact that plants are the only available, trusted medicine or the only affordable solution. As a result, plants continue to save millions of lives every year. Of the many plants used around the world, some have been carefully studied and used for the production of valuable drugs that can be found in pharmacies. Remarkably, of the hundreds of plant-derived pharmaceutical medicines, about 75% are used in modern medicine in ways correlating directly with their traditional uses by various native cultures! In other words, modern science has validated most of the traditional (should I say empirical? probably not) therapies involving plants. This remains valid for Moringa's precious medicinal properties, as we shall further explore.

How is Herbal Medicine Working?
How is Moringa Working?

Plants produce and contain thousands of chemical compounds that benefit the plant itself.

They protect the plant from herbivores or damaging ultraviolet light, attract pollinators or prevent competitive germination. Below are some examples of plant chemicals with biological activity in animals:

- Powerful alkaloids (alkaline reaction in water, contain nitrogen in their molecule) with specific actions on animal physiology. Caffeine (from coffee beans) and morphine (from poppy) are well known alkaloids. Moringa root bark, but not the rest of the plant, contains specific alkaloids such as moringinine, which increase heart and blood vessel tonus.

- Antioxidant compounds (please, refer to the chapter "Antioxidants in Moringa") reduce the cellular damage inflicted by normal metabolism and living processes in plants, animals, and humans. Most plant antioxidants are also anti-inflammatory and cancer-preventive, thus delaying aging of tissues, and degenerative diseases (age-related ailments). Examples of antioxidants are the compounds called flavonoids (color pigments found in many plants). To date, Moringa is known to contain a number of powerful antioxidant flavonoids such as quercetin and kaempferol. Many vitamins in Moringa qualify as potent antioxidants as well: vitamins A (as beta-carotene), C and E. (Please review "Antioxidants in Moringa.")

Dietary plants are the main source of antioxidant, antiaging substances for humans!

- **Vitamins** are complex substances vitally important for metabolic and many other physiological reactions. Some of the vitamins (specifically, vitamins A, C, E) are also potent antioxidants. Vitamins may be considered nutrients but they are also viewed as "medicines" when they bring the health back into balance, normalize and regulate the abnormal biologic processes which lead to diseases. Moringa is a powerful vitamin factory; some of those present in the various parts of the plant include vitamin C, beta-carotene (a precursor of vitamin A), vitamin E, vitamin K, and many of the B complex group of vitamins. These are reviewed extensively in the chapter "Moringa, the Nutritive Plant".

- **Antibiotics,** antimicrobial and antihelmintic (i.e., against parasites, worms) substances. Some of the most powerful antibiotics have been isolated from plants, but plants can also be used in their whole form to fight infections and parasite infestations. This extraordinary effect of plants is especially important whenever the local population cannot afford expensive medicines from pharmacies. Moringa has long been known to have powerful antibiotic effects and was used by various populations around

the globe against infections. Modern science
has confirmed and described at least some
of the antibiotic substances in Moringa. For
example, pterygospermin, a substance from her
flowers and roots, has excellent antimicrobial
and fungicidal properties. But that may not be
all; Moringa seeds and leaves might contain
antibiotic substances, yet to be discovered. Why
do I believe that? Because this plant, especially
the leaf juice, was traditionally used and is used
to treat many skin infections.

• **Natural hormones, enzymes, minerals,
  and various phytochemicals** (plant-derived
  substances) with numerous pharmacological
  activities in animals and humans. These are too
  numerous to mention, and they go beyond the
  purpose of this book to talk about their effects
  on health. Suffice it to say that plants, generally,
  are an inexhaustible, fantastically useful and
  creative source of beneficial substances that can
  be used in many ways to improve human lives, at
  all levels.

Niaziminin, another Moringa phytochemical,
was shown to have potent anticancer activity in
animal studies. Interestingly, long before research
validated the idea, people traditionally have used
Moringa against abdominal and other tumors
(cancerous growths).

Hypotensive (lower blood pressure) principles niazinin, niazimicin, and niaziminin A and B were also obtained from fresh leaves. These compounds belong to the family of mustard-oil glycosides (very rare in nature).

One of the most exciting phytochemicals found in Moringa is beta-sitosterol. It has a chemical structure very similar to that of cholesterol, and it acts to reduce the excess of cholesterol in the human blood. Although beta-sitosterol is not well absorbed by the body after ingestion, when consumed with cholesterol (found in animal fats) it effectively blocks cholesterol's absorption. This ultimately leads to a lower serum cholesterol level. But beta-sitosterol has many other beneficial effects for humans. Please review the chapter "Moringa, the Nutritive Plant" for more exciting details.

Moringa is rich in beneficial substances, hence her numerous pharmacological and nutritive activities. Her leaves are used for stabilizing blood pressure and blood sugar, plus reducing high levels of cholesterol in the blood. The pods are used to treat inflammations of the joints; the roots for rheumatism; the seeds have antispasmodic properties; the bark can be chewed to stimulate digestion; the flowers can heal various inflammations, and so on.

For a short summary of traditional, medicinal applications of Moringa, see Table 1.

IMPORTANT: It is worth mentioning that more often than not, it is impossible to point to a single, specific pharmacological effect of any particular phytochemical from a whole plant. Whole plants or their parts include a wide variety of active compounds that may act synergistically (complement and empower each other) or annihilate each other's unpleasant effects. The result of such multiple interactions between plant components, on one hand, and plant components and animal organisms (cells, tissues, organs) on the other hand, is expectedly complex. Humans (and animals!) have tried various plants and noticed their effects on overall health. These are, after all, time-tested medicines. Had they not helped healing, people would have discarded them and searched for other, more efficient plant medicines. In other words, if various cultures, in separate and distant parts of the world, have continued using Moringa as a medicinal plant, there must be very reliable beneficial effects.

Table 1 explores some of the best described healing properties of Moringa's seeds, leaves, and pods around the globe, from local traditional medicine. I wish to remind you that these medicinal applications, found and time-tested mostly in tropical and sub-tropi-cal regions, were made by people suffering from diseases generally different from those diseases of people in the developed world. Their main health concerns were various infections and parasites, malnourishment, and skin inflammations. High cholesterol, heart disease, cancers, and Alzheimer's disease were not on their priority list! But, as already mentioned and to be further explored, Moringa has plenty of healthy surprises for people with a wide variety of habits and problems.

A diet rich in plants such as Moringa can significantly improve human health by:

- Reducing cholesterol levels and triglycerides ("bad" fats in the serum).

- Controlling blood sugar and helping normal sugar and energy balance.

- Offering vitamins and minerals vital for maintaining normal physiology.

- Offering powerful antiaging and anti-inflammatory natural substances, many with anticancer properties.

Table 1

The Traditional Medicinal Uses of Some of Moringa's Parts by Various Cultures (African, Asian, American)

LEAVES	FLOWERS	PODS	SEEDS
general tonic	general tonic		tonic
anti-inflammatory	anti-inflammatory	anti-inflammatory	anti-inflammatory
anti-cancer	anti-cancer	anti-cancer	
diuretic	diuretic		treats bladder problems
antibacterial	antibacterial		antibacterial
antihelmintic[1]	antihelmintic	antihelmintic	
reduce fever	antibiotic		reduce fever
reduce headache			
laxative			laxative
anti-anemic			treat scurvy[2]
increase milk production			
anti-diarrheic			
antihypertensive			
anti-diabetic			
hepatoprotector			
relaxant sedative			

Note: Roots and bark are also used in a variety of ways for healing.

(1) Induce parasite eliminations (kills parasites and their eggs).

(2) A life-threatening disease due to deficiency of vitamin C.

It will beggar a doctor to live where orchards thrive.

Spanish proverb

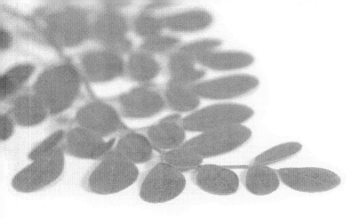

MORINGA,
THE NUTRITIVE PLANT

A more palatable subject, I hope, although nutrition and diet are pervasive buzz words that complicate our lives. Why? Because there is so much information (sometimes contradictory) and talk about food and nutrients, so many articles and shows everywhere you turn, that the subject leaves many people confused. It is not my wish to add more confusion to an otherwise important subject. Therefore I will explore Moringa's nutrients and benefits, while explaining briefly their role in human physiology.

What could Moringa bring to the Westerner's table?
Concentrated vitamins, minerals, all necessary protein constituents, beneficial fats, antioxidant, antiaging and anti-inflammatory substances, all in a readily absorbable form and easy to digest = an energy food. Tasty, but with very little sugar and salt.

First we saw the extraordinary benefits and nutritional value of Moringa for people living in less fortunate or impoverished areas which are prone to drought. The leaves, seeds and pods of Moringa provide many nutrients which can be eaten fresh or dried in a variety of recipes. According to Optima of Africa, Ltd. (optimaworld.com, a group that has been working with this tree in Tanzania), 25 grams (less than an ounce) daily of Moringa Leaf Powder "will give a child the following recommended daily allowances: **protein 42% , calcium 125%, magnesium 60%, potassium 41%, iron 71%, vitamin A 272%, vitamin C 22%.**" The same benefits apply to adults and senior citizens, but only the percentages change. Obviously, Moringa is beneficial for people of all ages.

It might seem hard to believe, but, despite the high frequency of obesity in our Western culture, many from the Western world suffer from serious nutritive deficiencies. They stem from poor eating habits (junk food, overcooking, mixing foods in an inappropriate way, etc.), insufficient consumption of fresh fruits, vegetables and seeds, foods lacking valuable nutrients due to soil depletion caused by intense, monoculture, chemically-laden methods of agriculture, or by over-processing of foods.

Many people, unknowingly, have poor gastro-in-testinal absorption of nutrients, which usually increases in seriousness with age. Many others lack

the time to learn about healthy nutrition, while
some are not educated enough to understand its
importance. Still others simply don't care, and stick
with their junk food until their first (or last) heart
attack.

Multivitamins (with minerals) seem to be
an easy and handy solution, but beware: many
vitamin brands offer pills and products that cannot
be truly dissolved and absorbed efficiently by the
body. They may also be contaminated with various
industrial substances (for example, solvents, heavy
metals, etc.). Generally, vitamins and most nutrients
are best absorbed and used by the body when
they come from natural sources (plants, animals)
and are present in naturally occurring, complex
combinations. This is because we humans ARE part
of the natural world. We evolved together with our
food for millions of years. Our digestive, metabolic,
and immune systems have been accustomed to
dealing with plants as a whole. We are designed to
best absorb vitamins from nature's complex foods.
So eat your veggies, whenever possible!

Summary of the Main Nutrients in *Moringa oleifera*

Most often leaves and pods of young shrubs
or adult plants are used for cooking. Sometimes
leaf powder (very concentrated in nutrients) may
be obtained for the convenience of handling and
transportation. There are already à number of
studies that have analyzed and measured the rich

variety of nutritive substances from Moringa. It is not my intention to overburden you with numbers and percentages, so I put together the following simplified Table 2 on page 30.

There are plenty of foods and treats on the market, each with more or less nutritive and caloric value. We try to make sense of them and choose the best, but what is "best"? For some, it is the taste, for others the vitamins, for many, the lack of cholesterol or sugar, or salt (strange, isn't it? - to value food for what it lacks.) There are thousands of books and opinions on food. Some get rich on the backs of others who, after reading those books, are still groping in the darkness of low calorie and low cholesterol, tasteless "health" bars.

Although, personally, I have been through medical schools and educational institutions in several countries, I can say my best and most reliable teacher is Nature! I take time to observe what Nature does, what animals that are like me eat or do; how healthy or sick they get, and what their secrets are for agility, energy, and longevity. I am not the only one. Ancient, wise civilizations did the same for thousands of years, observing and following Nature, in all details.

To make a long story short, I do what other omnivores like me do: eat a variety of fresh, non-cooked plants, mostly greens (lettuce, parsley, cabbage, spinach, and others), other colorful plants and fruits, seeds, nuts, mushrooms, and from time to time, some grains, eggs and lean meat (although I could live very well without meat). Since all these omnivores move a lot to collect those plants (think of the bear), I also move a lot. I think that is all you need to know about a healthy diet. Nature keeps things clear, simple and free of charge.

Coming back to Moringa - a green, most amazing and nutritious plant, I will describe the importance of her complex content in her characteristic, concentrated form (leaves or leaf powder and pods). Table 2 presents a brief summary of the main nutrients and other important components in Moringa for those who hate numbers and percentages.

Sometimes numbers are truly important since they enable us to compare nutritive values. So, for the sake of convincing the skeptics, let's look at some numbers, below.

Attention vegetarians and parents: In terms of protein value, the Moringa leaves are about 40% protein, with all of the 9 essential amino acids present in various amounts. (Essential amino acids are those that the human body cannot synthesize, therefore they must be supplied by the diet.) Moringa is considered to have the highest protein ratio of any plant so far studied on earth!

Attention lactose-intolerant friends: Calcium is a vital macroelement for human health. A cup (8 ounces) of milk or yogurt could supply 300-400 mg (about half of the daily necessary amount), while 8 ounces of Moringa leaves contain 1,000 mg calcium. Moringa leaf powder of the same weight (8 ounces) contains over 4,000 mg calcium.

Attention anemic friends: Moringa is very high in iron. Three ounces (about 100 g) contain 7 mg of iron, while the leaf powder has 28 mg. One of the richest iron sources, roast beef, has only 2 mg iron proportionally per three ounces.

Attention everybody: Vitamin C, one of the most disputed, talked about and supplemented vitamins, is found in Moringa in large quantities. 100 g of Moringa leaves contain more than 200 mg vitamin C, while 100 g of orange juice has only about 40 mg. The daily allowance…well, this is a long story that deserves more space, so we will meet again with this subject at the "Vitamin C" subchapter.

I know what you're thinking. All this sounds good, but who is going to replace the beef, oranges and yogurt with some leaves?

The answer is simple: the numbers and comparisons above were given for the purpose of evaluation and better appreciation of the extraordinary Moringa richness. I do not suggest you replace all of your favorites with "just" leaves. But, since most of us are concerned with calories while trying to nourish ourselves with nutrients and vitamins, Moringa can become a unique "super-food" in our arsenal. It is unique because, even in small amounts, it can supply daily a wide gamut of vital nutrients with few calories. It would take really large amounts and many types of foods - and calories - to bring all the nutrients, vitamins and minerals, antioxidants and antiaging substances we should eat every day. Why not add a concentrated super-food like Moringa? One plant has it all...even great taste!

For variety and simplicity in choices, parents concerned about their children's health should take a closer look at Moringa as a regular meal. Instead of supplying oranges for Vitamin C, milk for calcium, meat for iron and proteins, greens for magnesium, bananas for potassium, apples and pears for fiber, parents could use Moringa as a "Jack-of-All-Trades" regular snack.

Remember, VARIETY still remains the key for a healthy diet! I mean plant variety.

There are various sources for cooking and enjoying fresh Moringa leaves, pods or leaf powder. Please consult the references at the end of this book.

Table 2

The Main Nutritive Groups and Valuable Dietary Compounds in Moringa

1. Protein constituents or amino acids (the building blocks of proteins). There are 20 amino acids necessary, and found in human proteins, of which 9 are essential. ALL 9 are found in Moringa.

2. Carbohydrates (several of the "good" type, including fibers; about 3-13 % in pods and leaves).

3. Minerals as macroelements such as calcium, magnesium, potassium, phosphorus, sulfur.

4. Minerals as necessary microelements: iron, zinc, copper, manganese.

5. Fats, as vegetable oils: fatty acids, beneficial omega-6 oils and liposoluble vitamins.

6. Vitamins, many of which with antioxidant properties: Vitamin C, E, F, K, provitamin A (beta-carotene), complex of vitamins B—B1, B2, B3, choline, others.

7. Chlorophyll, the green pigment of plants (includes magnesium in its molecule).

8. Other plant pigments, some with antioxidant properties: lutein, carotenoids.

9. Plant hormones with antiaging properties in humans: cytokinins such as zeatin.

10. Plant specific (phytochemicals) antioxidants: quercetin, kaempferol and others.

11. Plant specific sterols: beta-sitosterol.

And many others beyond the scope of this book.

Amino Acids in Moringa

Plants are an important source of proteins, but most plants actually supply the units making up the proteins - the amino acids. As you know, proteins together with lipids and carbohydrates are the three basic groups of biochemical substances of which plant and animal organisms are made. Again, amino acids are the building blocks or monomers of the proteins (which are long chains of amino acids linked together).

How Much Protein Do We Need?

Nutrition experts recommend that proteins (or amino acids) should account for 10-15 % of the calories in a balanced diet, although requirements for protein are affected by age, health, weight, and other factors. Generally, a normal adult requires approximately 0.36 grams of protein per pound of body weight, or 0.8 grams per kg weight. That makes a total of 50-80 grams daily. Athletes have higher amino acid (protein) requirements, and babies need much more protein per body weight than do adults.

Proteins are digested by the gastro-intestinal system and then cut into smaller, simpler units (amino acids) that can be absorbed through the walls of the intestines and used by the body. After absorption, the liver and various tissues will make their own, specifically needed proteins. Thousands and thousands of complicated proteins make up the structure of cell walls, and the soluble particles in blood or less soluble structures of bone and skin. Proteins interact with each other and specifically recognize each other in order to perform ALL our physiological functions. Life can be seen as a complicated and beautiful "dance of proteins"! Since proteins and other nitrogen-containing substances are continuously degraded and rebuilt, they must be replaced by a continuous supply of amino acids from the diet.

Since proteins are cut into the smaller units and resynthesized afterwards, amino acids are the best material supply for making proteins in animals/ humans. By eating amino acids instead of long chains of proteins (as found in most animal-derived foods), the human body can save energy, time and... allergies. Many allergies are due to animal proteins. Therefore, by eliminating those proteins from one's diet, allergies can be treated or controlled efficiently. (Some allergies can also be due to plant proteins.) Since some babies are allergic to animal proteins or even soy proteins, they should be provided with amino acids, which are much smaller molecules, easier to absorb, and do not usually trigger allergies.

There are 20 amino acids present in the human body's structures. (Actually, in nature there are more amino acids.) Of those, 9 are known to be ESSENTIAL; they have to be supplied by the diet since the human body cannot synthesize them, as it does with the other 11 amino acids. Few foods, like Moringa, are known to contain all essential amino acids, hence, the importance of a complex, rich diet. The 9 essential amino acids are: histidine, isoleucine, leucine, lysine, methionine, phenylalanine, threonine, tryptophan and valine. Histidine is considered essential for children and babies, not for adults. Strict vegetarians should ensure that their diet contains sufficient amounts of all these amino acids.

Moringa is one of the very few plants that contain all the essential amino acids, although two of them, lysine and tryptophan, are poorly represented in most plants. Moringa's essential amino acids presence and digestibility scores are more than adequate when measured against the standards of WHO, Food and Agricultural Organization (FAO) and United Nations Organization (UNO) for small children, the most at-risk population group when it comes to proteins in food.

➤ Compared to soy beans, one of the best known and most valuable plant sources of proteins, Moringa's leaves fare great. The two plants have similar protein quality and quantity. Food scientists once believed that soy proteins were the only plant-based proteins with a quality equal to that of meat, milk and eggs, but now they have added Moringa to this very short list.

With all due respect to soy and its fans, I have to remind you that soy might be a wonderful source of proteins but it is not famous for its content of vitamin C, iron, calcium, and other nutrients. Moringa IS! Also, many babies are intolerant (allergic) to soy's protein. Sometimes these babies are lactose-intolerant as well, so they cannot drink milk or use it as a source of protein. Since there are no reports of any Moringa-trig-gered allergies, and since it is safely used as a food for numerous healthy and sick children, Moringa can become a principal source of amino acids in baby nutrition, replacing soy! *yes*

Another recent concern related to soy is that a large proportion of the soy cultivated in USA today is genetically modified (GM) but not labeled as such. The European Union, Japan and other countries often reject GM plants or require strict labeling of the foods containing GM products. Soy is present in a large variety of products, from baby food to supplements, in soy protein isolate or flour. Most believe that there is no safe way to identify and differentiate GM soy from non-GM soy in USA or Canada. While the debate about GM plants is very hot and understandably so, I do not intend to discuss this here. Suffice it to say that GM plants contain foreign proteins, sometimes derived from insects, that may induce allergies and other health problems in some people. GM plants also pose a serious threat for the environment and common plants or agricultural heritage. Their long-term effects on human health have not been studied yet, but GM plants have been highly promoted and sold unlabeled on North American food market shelves. Therefore, to vegetarians and everybody concerned about their plant protein sources, such as soy, Moringa's amino acids should be a first-line supply, together with her other wonderful nutritive qualities!

Table 3 compares the essential amino acids composition in Moringa and soy proteins. Don't miss this eye-opening table!

Table 3

Essential Amino Acids Composition in Proteins of Moringa (leaves) and Soy (protein isolate)

Essential Amino Acid	Soy Protein mg/g protein	FAO/WHO 2-5 year old child Reference Pattern mg/g protein	*Moringa oleifera* Extracted Leaves mg/g protein
Histidine	26	19	31
Isoleucine	49	28	51
Leucine	82	66	98
Lysine	63	58	66
Methionine + Cystine	26	25	21
Phenylalanine + Tyrosine	90	63	105
Threonine	38	34	50
Tryptophan	13	11	21
Valine	50	35	63

(*Moringa oleifera* amino acid values are taken from F. N. Makkar et al., see references. These values can vary slightly from product to product.)

In the following pages I will introduce the essential amino acids of Moringa and briefly explain their importance for human health. The majority of

North Americans eat more than enough protein and each of the essential amino acids. BUT dieters, strict vegetarians, and anyone consuming an inadequate number of calories may not ingest adequate amounts of essential amino acids. In the latter cases, the body will break down the proteins in the muscle and use those amino acids to meet the needs of vital organs. In cases of amino acid deficiency, especially in children, certain diseases and stunted growth might occur.

REMEMBER: as with all other nutrients, the amino acids are best absorbed from a complex, naturally-occurring food or plant source.

Histidine - Moringa leaves contain histidine, a semi-essential amino acid - adults generally produce adequate amounts but children usually may not. It is believed that histidine may increase the body's resistance to environmental toxins and allergens (factors that trigger allergies in susceptible persons). Since histidine is found abundantly in hemoglobin the respiratory pigment protein needed for oxygen transportation to every cell - histidine aids in the prevention of anemia.

Histidine is also a mild vasodilator and helps increase blood circulation. According to some research, people with rheumatoid arthritis have low levels of histidine; therefore it has been used in the treatment of rheumatoid arthritis. A deficiency of histidine can also cause poor hearing. Since histidine is found in numerous proteins, its presence is needed for normal general physiology.

Isoleucine - Moringa contains isoleucine in large amounts. Its main role in the body is related to its incorporation into many proteins and enzymes. This is one of the essential amino acids needed for hemoglobin formation, as is histidine. Therefore, its presence is useful for the prevention or treatment of anemia. Isoleucine plays a role in optimal growth during childhood; babies and children need much more isoleucine per body weight than adults! It also maintains normal blood sugar and energy levels and therefore it is particularly important for diabetics. Isoleucine is metabolized in muscle tissue and can enhance energy levels and increase endurance. Athletes and everyone exercising regularly need extra isoleucine.

Leucine - This is another essential amino acid related to isoleucine and valine, all vital for normal growth in children. Moringa contains large amounts of leucine as well. These three amino acids work together to protect muscles, build muscles, and enhance energy levels and stamina. They also promote bone, skin and muscle tissue healing and therefore are recommended for those recovering from injuries, stress or surgery. Leucine may help to lower elevated blood sugar levels, which is important for diabetics. For normal growth, small children and babies need much more leucine per body weight than adults. Leucine also aids in increasing growth hormone production.

Lysine - Lysine is required for normal growth and development in children, who need vast amounts of this amino acid. Although plant sources are usually poor in lysine, Moringa leaves are quite rich in this essential amino acid. Lysine helps calcium absorption and bone development, and maintains a proper protein balance. Lysine also aids in the production of antibodies (protective proteins of the immune system), hormones and enzymes, in skin maintenance and formation, and tissue repair. Since it helps to build muscle protein, lysine is necessary for those recovering from stress, injuries and surgery. In people with "bad" serum fats and high cholesterol, lysine lowers high serum triglyceride levels.

Another useful quality of lysine is its capacity to inhibit the multiplication of viruses, especially herpes viruses.

Methionine and Cystine - These are important sulfur-containing amino acids. Cystine is the stable form of the sulfur-containing amino acid **cysteine.** The body readily converts one into the other as needed, therefore the two forms can be considered as a single amino acid in metabolism. Sulfur-containing amino acids are involved in detoxification of the organism; they help to neutralize and eliminate harmful toxins and protect the body against radiation damage caused by UV rays and x-rays. They are free radical destroyers, and work best when taken with selenium and vitamin E (see "Antioxidants in Moringa"). Cystine helps to protect the liver and brain from damage due to toxics such as alcohol, drugs, and environmental pollutants.

Methionine and cystine are main constituents of the proteins of fingernails, skin and hair; they promote proper elasticity and texture of the skin and hair. Ladies, real beauty comes from the inside, and sulfur-containing amino acids must surely be ingredients of any diet that fights skin aging!

Cystine may have anti-inflammatory properties that can be helpful in the treatment of osteoarthritis and rheumatoid arthritis. Cystine and methionine are recommended to be supplemented in the treatment of some forms of cancer. These two amino acids also promote wound healing; therefore they are helpful after surgery and burns. They are known to bind iron, aiding in iron absorption. For those interested in losing weight, it is worth mentioning that cystine also promotes the burning of fat and the building of muscle.

Phenylalanine and Tyrosine - These two essential amino acids, well represented in Moringa leaves, are particularly important for the health of the central nervous system. Once in the body, phenylalanine can be converted into tyrosine, which in turn is used to synthesize two key brain transmitters that promote alertness: dopamine and norepinephrine. These two amino acids - phenylalanine and tyrosine - can therefore elevate mood, decrease pain, help with memory and even suppress appetite.

Phenylalanine and tyrosine should be supplemented in the treatment of depression, arthritis, obesity and Parkinson's disease. Phenylalanine is effective for controlling pain, especially the chronic pain in osteoarthritis and rheumatoid arthritis, according to some studies. Similar to other amino acids, these two are incorporated in a variety of proteins throughout the body.

Threonine - Threonine is also very well represented in Moringa, although its content is usually low in many grains and other plant protein sources. This amino acid is important for the formation of collagen and elastin, two main proteins of the skin. It also helps to protect the liver and has a lipotropic function (against fatty liver). Threonine is present in high concentrations in the proteins of the heart, central nervous system and skeletal muscle. It maintains their health and normal functions. It also enhances the immune system by aiding in the production of antibodies, and promotes thymus (a gland vital for the function of the immune system) growth and related activity. Other vital nutrients are also better absorbed when threonine is present in the food. Some use threonine supplements in certain cases of depression. Infants need much more (8 times) threonine per body weight than adults.

Tryptophan - An essential amino acid, tryptophan is required for the production of niacin (vitamin B3) and serotonin (the neurotransmitter involved in relaxation and sleep) among others. Therefore, tryptophan helps to control depression and insomnia, stabilizes emotional moods, and it also eases perception of pain, and might combat inflammation. It also aids to control hyperactivity in children and alleviates stress. Although tryptophan is the rarest of all amino acids to be found in protein's composition, it plays an important role in reducing stress-related mood disorders, and helps relaxation and good sleep! We all need some extra tryptophan sometimes! Supplements of tryptophan are not approved in the USA, so, when needed, we have to get it from food. Moringa is an excellent plant source of tryptophan, and its concentration in the leaves exceeds the concentration in soy beans. Since some migraine sufferers have abnormally low levels of tryptophan, it is believed that tryptophan can also ease the pains associated with certain types of migraines.

Valine - Unlike tryptophan, valine has a stimulant effect. It is needed for muscle metabolism and structure, general tissue repair and the maintenance of a proper protein balance in the body. Valine is found in high concentrations in muscles, similar to related amino acids, isoleucine and leucine. These three branched-chain amino acids can be used as an energy source by muscle tissue, thus preserving the use of glucose and supplying stamina. Studies have shown that these amino acids are useful in restoring muscle mass in people with liver disease, or after physical stress, injuries and surgery. Moringa leaves are at least as rich (if not more) as soy beans (and soy protein concentrate) in valine.

SUMMARY

Moringa is one of the very few plant sources that contain all 9 essential amino acids.

Moringa's essential amino acids presence and digestibility are as good as soy (one of the best protein sources). Soy is often a highly processed product while Moringa is presented in its natural state.

Moringa's essential amino acids presence and digestibility are better than those required by the standards of WHO, FAO and UNO. Moringa, even in small portions, provides adequate amounts of protein nutrients for everyone, including healthy or medically compromised individuals, children, senior adults, lactose intolerant individuals, vegetarians and people with soy allergies.

Moringa is not genetically modified or altered by humans.

Moringa is considered to have the highest protein ratio of any plant so far identified!

Minerals in Moringa

Our bodies contain, in various amounts, about 5% minerals. Over 20 minerals are known to be needed for normal physiology - some in relatively large amounts (known as macroelements), such as calcium, potassium, and phosphorus, and others in small amounts (known as microelements or trace minerals), like iron, copper and zinc. Some believe that we have in our bodies all the minerals of our planet, and they all play a role, although not entirely understood by scientists at this time. Research continues!

For simplification, minerals have two general functions: building tissues and regulating their function. Almost every process in our bodies is regulated at one level or another by minerals. Consequently, together with proteins, carbohydrates, fats and vitamins, we must ingest a proper amount of minerals for health maintenance.

The human body does not produce minerals; they all must be provided by food!

Macroelements in Moringa

Moringa leaves, pods, flowers, and seeds contain varying amounts of important macroelements such as calcium, magnesium, potassium, phosphorus and sodium.

Calcium

Moringa leaves contain high amounts of calcium, about 500 mg per 100 g of leaves, while the leaf powder can have about five times more calcium per 100 g. The daily recommended dose for an adult is about 1,000 mg, with more needed for pregnant or lactating women. Remember, calcium is consumed and excreted every day. Ideally and importantly, the consumed calcium should equal the amount of calcium excreted.

Calcium is a vital mineral for numerous physiological processes, such as building and maintaining healthy bones and teeth, blood clotting and other various cellular functions (maintaining normal heart rhythm and the transmission of nerve impulses). Almost all the calcium in the human body is stored in the bones and teeth, and when calcium is needed in the blood (for instance, if it is missing from the diet for a while), it is released (borrowed) from bones. This can lead to decalcification of bones if extended over long periods of time. Calcium is important for so many body functions, yet most of us associate calcium only with bone health or disease. Let's explore the role of calcium in maintaining strong bones.

Bones are living tissues, constantly formed and remodeled. Even in healthy individuals (who get enough calcium and physical activity), bone destruction exceeds bone production after the age of 30. Osteoporosis (porous bones), another buzz word today, is caused by an imbalance between bone building (less active) and bone destruction (excessive). More than ten million Americans (mostly menopausal women) have osteoporosis.

How Can We Delay or Prevent Osteoporosis?

The answer is by eating adequate amounts of calcium and maximizing bone stores during the times when bone is growing fast - especially up to age 30!

- By exercising regularly.
- By consuming adequate amounts of vitamin K, usually found in green leaves.
- By getting enough vitamin D.

Moringa benefits here in at least two ways; by its high content of calcium and by its good content of vitamin K. But, as we shall see later, Moringa, as a plant, may fight osteoporosis in other ways, as well.

We can obtain calcium from various food sources including dairy products (with high concentration of absorbable calcium) and dark leafy greens or beans (with varying amounts of absorbable calcium). There is a hot debate over which source is actually better for supplying calcium that can be utilized by the bones and used by the whole body.

According to recent research, too much animal protein intake can leach calcium from the bones. As the body digests protein, it releases acids into the bloodstream, which are neutralized by drawing calcium from the bones. The more animal proteins, the more acidity in the body, the less calcium in the bones. It is clear now that animal proteins can cause more acidity and calcium leaching from the bones than plant proteins. Plants, or a plant-based diet actually alkalinize the body, while animal proteins acidify the body. These facts might also explain why certain people who consume much less animal products (including milk and cheese) suffer significantly less osteoporosis than North Americans or Europeans. Good plant sources of calcium (such as Moringa) are better for long term prevention of calcium loss!

Are there any other reasons for supplying your calcium mostly from plant sources?

You bet!

1. Dairy products are high in "bad" saturated fats that increase the risk of heart disease and other illnesses.

2. Many people including Asians, Hispanics, African Americans and especially children have lactose intolerance.

3. Galactose (a milk sugar) has been linked with a high incidence of ovarian problems, including cancer.

The following table (Table 4) compares the approximate amounts of calcium in various sources, both of animal and plant origins.

Table 4

Comparison of Various Calcium-rich Food Sources	
Food (100g)	**Calcium (mg)**
Skimmed milk	120
Yogurt, low fat	180
Spinach	130
Cheese	480
Beans	60
Iceberg lettuce	90
Salmon	180
Nuts, seeds	70
Green peas	35
Moringa leaves	**440**

Magnesium

Moringa leaves and pods contain another important macroelement, magnesium; approximately 25 mg per 100 g of leaves or pods, while the leaf powder can contain approximately 370 mg per the same weight.

Magnesium is similar to calcium in several ways; 60% is found in the bones and teeth, and the balance is found mostly in the muscles. Magnesium is the second-most abundant positively charged element found within the cells, where it plays vital roles in the processing of energy. Magnesium is linked to a substance known as adenosine tri-phosphate, or ATP, the main "energy molecule" in the body, which activates about 300 different enzymes and enzymatic reactions involved in functions such as genetic material synthesis, energy storage, intracellular mineral transport, muscle contraction, nerve transmission, blood vessel tone, and many others. Magnesium is extremely vital to health as:

- It stimulates gastric motility and intestinal function (it is a laxative).

- It is a relaxing ion for the nervous system and blood vessels; thus it fights stress, irritability, and high blood pressure.

- It is involved in calcium metabolism and bone fixation; therefore magnesium supplementation improves bone mineral density, while low intake has been associated with the development of osteoporosis.

- It has an important role in lung structure and function.

The recommended dietary dose for magnesium is 350 mg per day for men and 280 milligrams for women. Magnesium is obtained from the diet, but not all sources are equal in terms of bioavailability. How much magnesium is truly absorbed and used by the body? Magnesium derived from metallic sources (such as salts of magnesium present in water or many vitamin pills) is less absorbable, whereas magnesium derived from plant sources is more easily absorbed.

ATTENTION SOFT DRINK LOVERS: The excess phosphate found in soft drinks depletes your magnesium; therefore you need higher amounts than recommended. This is also valid for over-stressed people (hmm...like me and you), athletes, pregnant and lactating women, and diabetics. Long-term magnesium deficiency may manifest as depression, irritability, heart problems, weakness, poor coordination, nausea, vomiting, and tremors.

Diets including plenty of fruits and greens (which are good sources of magnesium) are consistently associated with lower blood pressure, lower risk of coronary heart disease, and stroke.

Potassium

Potassium, another beneficial mineral, is high in both Moringa leaves and powder. Moringa leaves and pods contain about 260 mg of potassium per 100 g of leaves or pods, while the leaf powder can have approximately 1,300 mg per same weight. Another beneficial thing about Moringa is that it is low in sodium. The ideal ratio between these two ions, sodium and potassium, should be 1:1. Unfortunately, most Westerners have diets too high in sodium and too low in potassium. Processed foods usually add sodium but not potassium. Moringa would bring more potassium than sodium into your diet. The adult potassium recommended intake is approximately 2-3 g daily.

What Does Potassium Do in the Body?

- It is involved in nerve and brain functions, muscle control and blood pressure. Potassium lowers blood pressure, acting as an antagonist of sodium.

- It works with sodium to maintain the water balance, which is very important for good health.

- It assists in the regulation of the acid-base balance and water balance in the blood.

- It assists in protein synthesis from amino acids, and in carbohydrate metabolism.

Potassium is vital for health, but supplementation should never be taken without the approval of a healthcare provider! Too much potassium, taken too fast, is dangerous for the heart. But plant sources are not as dangerous from this point of view, as multivitamins and mineral supplements are. So, eat green!

Moringa (100 g leaves or 25 g leaf powder) is an excellent concentrated source of potassium. Here's how Moringa compares with the following foods that provide 200-400 mg of potassium per portion:

Milk	- 1 cup
Spinach	- ½ cup
Broccoli	- ½ cup
Tomato	- 1 (large)

Phosphorus

Moringa contains phosphorus, an important mineral which serves as the main regulator of energy metabolism in cells. As you know, it is also important for bone and teeth health. It also helps the body absorb glucose (a type of carbohydrate found in foods as well as in our blood), and transport fatty acids. Phosphorous, in various types of salts, is part of the buffer system that maintains the normal acid-base balance of the body. Moringa contains about 100 mg of phosphorus in 100 g of leaves, while the leaf powder contains twice as much.

Sulfur

Now this is the Cinderella of all minerals. Sulfur is one of the most important but neglected nutrients, maybe more important than magnesium, iron, sodium, iodine and even many vitamins. Sulfur has incredibly diverse roles; it is part of many proteins, boosts resistance to diseases, regulates blood sugar and helps detoxify the body. Sulfur is the third most abundant mineral, after calcium and phosphorus, in the body, but researchers have not yet established the exact daily requirement. It is assumed we all get enough sulfur IF we eat plenty of proteins or other compounds containing this element - mostly in fresh or non-cooked foods. (Most people are sulfur deficient unless they eat fish and raw meat and their vegetables uncooked!) Most of us need about 850 mg of sulfur for basic turnover (exchange rate or daily needs to replace what was used in the body). Moringa offers a good quantity and quality of organic, absorbable sulfur, from 140 mg per 100 g of leaves and pods, to more than 800 mg in 100 g leaf powder, making it an excellent source of sulfur for everyone.

Why is Sulfur So Important?

Sulfur is found in every living cell; it is a constituent of the essential amino acids methionine and cysteine, vitamins B1 and biotin (another type of B vitamin), the powerful antioxidant glutathione (see below) and the anticoagulant heparin. Sulfur is found in hormones like insulin, which regulates blood glucose levels. Sulfur is part of the biological "cement" that keeps cells and tissues together, forms skin, hair, nails and the cartilage that pads the joints. Now it aches! We would fall apart without sulfur.

Glutathione is composed of the three amino acids cysteine (containing sulfur), glycine and glutamic acid (two non-essential amino acids). Glutathione is one of the most powerful antioxidants made by the human body. Low levels of glutathione are associated with heart disease and cancer. In addition, it also helps the liver detoxify dangerous chemicals of all sorts. More than 90% of the non-protein-bound sulfur in the cells is found as glutathione.

Speaking about pain and joints, many are now familiar with the sulfur-based compound MSM or methylsulfonylmethane, a natural substance present in humans, many animals and certain plants. MSM is 34 percent sulfur. MSM is so important for pain and inflammation relief (in arthritis, back pain, headaches, fibromyalgia and others), that is now present in various supplements. You can help your body produce this beneficial sulfur-containing substance right there where it is needed. The sulfur from uncooked Moringa can be absorbed and used to synthesize the necessary sulfur-containing substances. Be good to your joints and get your sulfur from organic sources. It could help alleviate those joint pains!

Microelements in Moringa

Last, but not least of the minerals, microelements are called "micro" not because they are of less importance, but because they are needed in smaller amounts than macroelements such as calcium. Moringa contains significant amounts of microelements such as iron, zinc, copper, manganese and selenium. I am sure, as the research on Moringa progresses, more minerals will be discovered in the plant.

Iron

Moringa is already famous for her high content of this vital mineral. I don't know if Popeye has yet found out, but Moringa has much more iron than spinach. 100 g of leaves or pods, or 25 g (less than an ounce) of leaf powder could provide all the daily iron needs of an adult, about 10-20 mg. Iron deficiency is a serious problem not only in impoverished regions of the world, but even in the USA. A recent United States Department of Agriculture (USDA) survey indicated that small children (1-2 years old) and women ages 12-49 do not get enough iron for their physiological needs from their diets! Surprised?

Iron is one of those finicky nutrients that like good company in order to be absorbed and stay in your body! While many foods contain iron, it is not easily absorbed unless certain nutrients such as vitamin C and others are present. Iron in animal foods, such as meat, is well absorbed (15-45 %) but is not well absorbed from dairy products, or grains (including your breakfast cereals!). Coffee, red wine and black tea also inhibit the absorption of iron from food, while multi-vitamin/ multi-mineral pills do not really help you with iron, either. Remember, I mentioned earlier the importance of ingesting complex foods rather than taking vitamin pills for the best source of nutrients? Since Moringa contains high amounts of vitamin C (please review "Vitamins in Moringa"), it represents an excellent source of absorbable iron.

Why is Iron So Important?

Iron is a constituent of the main protein that carries oxygen in the blood to all cells - hemoglobin - and also forms part of the oxygen-carrying protein myoglobin in the muscles. As you know, our bodies cannot function without oxygen being transported to all tissues. Iron is also a necessary component of many enzymes, the dynamic proteins involved in all metabolic, digestive and respiratory processes. Iron is concentrated in storage forms in the body, as ferritin and hemosiderin (15 % of the iron is stored for future needs and mobilized when food intake is inadequate). Women with heavy menstrual periods can lose significant amounts of iron. Too much iron is not good either; consequently the body strives to maintain normal iron levels by controlling the amount of iron absorbed from food. Supplements in the form of soluble iron salts can be dangerous if there is no iron deficiency. Again, the best source of iron is your nutritious food!

Zinc

Another essential mineral found in almost every cell in small amounts, zinc stimulates the activity of more than 100 enzymes. As I mentioned above, enzymes are substances that catalyze (accelerate) and promote a multitude of biochemical reactions in the body. Zinc supports a healthy immune system, wound healing, normal growth and development during pregnancy, childhood and adolescence. It is also needed for genetic material synthesis. Zinc, similar to iron, is found in a variety of foods, in different quantities, with different degrees of absorbability. Moringa leaves, pods and seeds contain zinc in amounts similar to those found in beans, while the leaf powder has twice as much zinc per the same weight.

Copper

Believe it or not, we also need copper! All the copper found in the body (80-120 mg) would fit on the head of a pin, nevertheless, it is known that copper is vital for optimal health. While copper is found everywhere in the body, it is concentrated in organs with high metabolic activity such as liver, heart and brain (copper is crucial for the normal development of the nervous system). Copper plays a role in the synthesis and maintenance of myelin, a substance which insulates nerve cells to ensure proper transmission of nerve impulses, and as a cofactor for processes that neutralize the dangerous free radicals that would otherwise destroy our cells. We would not be able to produce energy without the help of copper and co-helper enzymes. Healthy muscles, including the heart, could not work without copper. Proper skin appearance and properties, and bone formation also require copper.

Hmm, all these statistics make you consider chewing some pennies...well, copper is also found in Moringa. One hundred grams of leaves provide enough copper for the daily allowance in an adult (about 1 mg). People living on a highly refined or over-processed diet, as many Westerners are, need more copper. Refined foods, meat and dairy products are generally lower in copper than diets rich in vegetables and unrefined grains.

Manganese

This is another essential trace mineral with multiple functions. Manganese is mostly concentrated in the bones, liver, pancreas and brain. It is a component of several enzymes such as manganese-superoxide dismutase, which prevents tissue damage due to oxidation. Manganese also activates numerous enzymes involved in the digestion and utilization of foods, breakdown of cholesterol, sex hormone production and the function of bones and skin.

The estimated adequate dietary intake for manganese is 2-5 mg for adults. Moringa has 5 mg per 100 g leaves or 50 g leaf powder, and thus qualifies as an outstanding source of manganese. In humans, manganese deficiencies are rare, although some groups of population might have suboptimal levels (including people with osteoporosis and multiple sclerosis). Moringa sources are better than many others considered excellent (providing more than 1 mg manganese per serving) including pecans, peanuts, oatmeal and bran cereal. Attention, very little manganese is found in meat or fish, dairy products or sweet and refined foods! Please read food labels! See what you eat and notice how many vital nutrients are missing or are low in processed, cooked foods.

Selenium

Selenium is an essential trace element with powerful antioxidant properties. For more detailed information on this particular beneficial property of selenium, please review "Antioxidants in Moringa". This mineral also functions as a component of enzymes involved in thyroid hormone metabolism. Medical research has shown that increased selenium intake decreases the risk of many types of cancers including breast, colon, lung and prostate cancers. Selenium also preserves tissue elasticity, slows down the aging of tissues (through its antioxidant properties) and even helps in the treatment of dandruff.

The daily selenium need for adults is 50 -70 mcg (micrograms; one mcg represents one thousandth of a mg). Vegetal foods (fruits and vegetables) generally provide little selenium, but Moringa contains about 8-10 mcg per 100 g leaf powder.

SUMMARY

Moringa has a substantial content of vital macro and microelements such as calcium, iron and sulfur, all absolutely necessary for good health.

Humans do not produce minerals; therefore, they all must be provided from food.

Moringa leaves contain calcium in quantities similar to cheese, and far higher than most plants.

Moringa leaves are very rich in iron in comparison with spinach and other plants.

Moringa also contains important microelements such as manganese and selenium.

"The tree which moves some to tears of joy is in the eyes of others only a green thing that stands in the way. Some see Nature all ridicule and deformity, and some scarce see Nature at all. But to the eyes of the man of imagination, Nature is Imagination itself."

William Blake, 1799 - "The Letters"

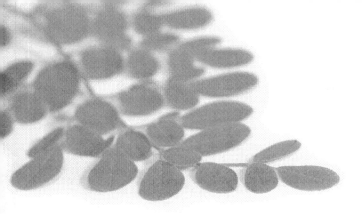

FATS IN MORINGA

Moringa seeds contain between 30-42% oil, with 13% saturated fats and 82% unsaturated fatty acids (those considered very beneficial in the diet). The leaves and pods, surprisingly, also contain 1-2% fats. Since Moringa is a food champion and seems to gather all the best nutrients for us, don't be surprised to find out that it also provides some of the absolutely essential fats or Essential Fatty Acids (EFA's), and other "good" fats as oils. (As in the case of essential amino acids, the EFA's cannot be naturally synthesized by the human body therefore they must be obtained from the diet.) *Moringa oleifera* (oleifera is the Latin term for "oil-containing") surely deserves her name.

The Good, the Bad and the ...Oleic Acid.

Don't eat too much fat! A fatty diet is unhealthy, right? WRONG!

Fats of the good sort, as we shall further explore, are absolutely vital for health. All cells, especially the membranes surrounding the cells, contain large amounts of fats (including cholesterol), and our brains are composed mostly of fat. Can't keep a brain without fat! Most of the body's biology (including heart function, blood pressure, fertility, inflammation and immunity-resistance to various infections and even cancer) depends on the presence of optimal fats. Damaged cells are replaced with new ones on a daily basis; in this process, fats are absolutely necessary as they make up a good proportion of the cell membranes.

A low-fat diet will make you very ill in the long run; it induces heart problems, stunts growth, harms the liver, kidneys, endocrine glands (that secrete our hormones) and the immune system (that protects us against infections and cancer).

Not all fats are equal, though. While animal sources contain mostly saturated fats (more hydrogen in their chemical structure) - or "bad" fats, many plant-derived fats are high in unsaturated, beneficial oils. The more unsaturated a fat is, the more liquid (oily).

What about the amount of fats in the diet? Detailed research has shown that the total amount of fat in the diet (high or low) isn't really linked with disease, but what really matters is the **type** of fat in the diet. The secret is to substitute good, vegetable fats for bad fats.

> Saturated fats increase the occurrence of chronic diseases, inflammations, heart problems, strokes, atherosclerosis and others.
>
> Unsaturated fats protect against many diseases, including cancer, nourish the body and fight inflammation, depression and infections.

A particularly harmful group of fats are the man-synthesized hydrogenated (trans) fats that can be found in everything today, such as biscuits and candies, margarines and vegetable shortening, fast foods and in most commercially baked goods.

What About Cholesterol in Food?

Although it is important to limit the amount of cholesterol in the diet, dietary cholesterol isn't the main enemy. High cholesterol in the bloodstream may significantly increase the risk for heart disease and strokes. But the cholesterol in the blood is mostly (75 %) made in the liver, while only a quarter is derived from what is absorbed from food. Again, the biggest influence on blood cholesterol level is the ratio and type of fats in the diet. (For more information about cholesterol and why Moringa could help, please review the chapter "Beta-sitosterol in Moringa".)

One of the best types of fats is oleic acid, a monounsaturated oil which is actually present in Moringa in high quantities. About 73% of the Moringa oil is oleic acid, while in most beneficial plant oils, it only contributes up to 40%! For instance, olive oil (one of the best, most healthy types of fats) is about 75% oleic acid, while sunflower is about 20%, and canola about 55% oleic acid. Similar to olive oil, Moringa has only 13% saturated fats.

You must have heard about oleic acid, the main fat in olive oil - one of the best known secrets of the healthy Mediterranean diet, which is linked to lower rates of cardiovascular disease and certain types of cancer. The Mediterranean diet is actually rich in fats, but we are really talking about the good oleic acid. Science has clearly established the link between reduced incidence of cardiovascular disease and olive oil (oleic acid) and it is believed that this is due to its ability to lower cholesterol levels. (High cholesterol levels are a main risk factor for cardiovascular disease.) Risk factors of heart disease, stroke and high blood pressure, are also positively affected by oleic acid. Some scientists have recommended the daily use of olive oil to lower the need for antihypertensive drugs! Oleic acid also reduces atherosclerosis (hardening of the arteries). European studies have found significantly lower breast cancer incidence among women with a high intake of monounsaturated fats, mainly in the form of olive oil. As of this date, science has yet to study the benefits of Moringa oil, but that date will surely come in the not too distant future. However, since Moringa oil is so similar to olive oil, one could expect similar beneficial properties.

Another exciting property of oleic acid is related to its ability to regulate the blood glucose levels. Glucose is the common type of sugar in the blood. Research studies have shown that olive oil can markedly lower blood glucose levels. Even diabetics who switch from a high carbohydrate/ low fat diet to a high fat (50% of calories coming from fat) diet, with most of that fat as olive oil, can lower their blood sugar levels so much that they require less insulin injections. Insulin is the pancreatic hormone regulating, among others, the blood glucose levels. Some diabetics do not produce enough insulin anymore, others have become "insulin resistant" - meaning that their cells do not recognize and do not react anymore to the body's own insulin. Both groups require constant treatment and careful diet habits. Even in the case of insulin resistance, oleic acid may help to prevent or delay the onset of the diabetes by preventing insulin resistance. Many overweight people are candidates for diabetes with insulin resistance. For them and for anybody else, it is worth taking a good look at oleic acid and replacing the saturated fats with plant oils rich in oleic acid.

Similar to olive oil, Moringa oil also contains 1-2 % EFA's such as the omega 3 and omega 6. EFA's favorably affect atherosclerosis, coronary heart disease, inflammatory disease, depression and even behavioral disorders (temper tantrums, learning, and hyperactivity in children).

An inadequacy of essential fatty acids is one of the main, widespread nutritional deficiencies among Americans and, generally, other modern societies consuming a refined or over-processed diet. This is a serious health risk, especially for children, since fatty acids are crucial for proper growth. *The brain development of growing fetuses and newborns depends absolutely on the presence of EFA's.*

ATTENTION PARENTS OF HYPERACTIVE CHILDREN: Recent studies have shown that hyperactive children have much lower levels of essential fatty acids! Take a look at the labels of the cookies, cereals, peanut butter and other foods - replace foods containing hydrogenated or trans fats, and introduce instead plenty of good, fresh fats: raw nuts, extra virgin olive oil, flax, fish and...Moringa!

<u>SUMMARY</u>

Moringa oil fat composition is very similar to that
of olive oil, one of the most studied, most beneficial
types of fat.

The main (73 %) fat in Moringa—oleic acid—is
an unsaturated fat linked to reduced incidence of
heart disease, neurological disease, atherosclerosis,
infections, and various cancers.

Moringa leaves and seeds also contain beneficial
essential fatty acids (EFA's).

The type of fat is more important than the amount of
fat in the diet.

Strive for Unsaturated Fats!

"Trees are sanctuaries. Whoever knows how to speak to them, whoever knows how to listen to them, can learn the truth. They do not preach learning and precepts, they preach undeterred by particulars, the ancient law of life."

Hermann Hesse — "Wandering"

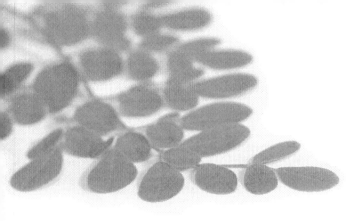

VITAMINS IN MORINGA

No Cinderella here, all these wonderfully beneficial substances, known as vitamins, have been thoroughly studied and described. However, I am sure we will keep on discovering new exciting things about them. Moringa is a vitamin treasure. Vitamins C, E, F, K, provitamin A (beta-carotene), many of the complex of vitamins B - B1, B2, B3 and choline -are found in various parts of Moringa.

What Are Vitamins?

Vitamins are organic compounds absolutely essential for growth and maintenance of life in plants and animals. They are classified into two groups:

- Fat-soluble (liposoluble) - vitamins A, D, E, K. These may be stored in the body in fat tissues.

- Water-soluble (hydro-soluble) - the B complex, vitamin C. These are excreted when not needed for use. Replenishment of these to the body is a critical process.

Interestingly, vitamins have the same roles in almost all forms of life, but higher animals (including humans) have lost the capacity to synthesize many of them. Consequently, most vitamins have to be supplied by food. Vitamin deficiency generates serious diseases in all organisms requiring them.

What functions do vitamins perform? Vitamins function in many metabolic reactions. For instance, fat-soluble vitamins act as regulators of specific metabolic reactions, while water-soluble vitamins function as coenzymes (workmates of enzymes which control biochemical reactions and utilization of energy). Important biological functions such as blood coagulation, vision, growth and development, tissue structuring and connectivity, bone formation and calcium fixation, and many others depend on the presence of appropriate amounts of vitamins.

There is so much information available about vitamins (often contradictory) that it seems that anyone can be a specialist. Multivitamin pills are in every household today, although it is safe to say that most people in the Western world probably do not need multivitamins regularly. Of course, a medical prescription is an exception. In addition, many suppliers offer vitamins that are not truly absorbed due to poor formulations. These vitamins are not truly "bioavailable" (absorbable and available for maximum effectiveness to the body). Alternatively, all humans need complex, natural vitamins provided by a nutritious diet consisting mostly of plants (leaves, fruits, seeds, roots, sprouts, legumes, mushrooms, etc.). Remember, nutrients are meant to work in a delicate balance with each other, not as separate compounds, as often formulated in pills, capsules and tablets.

Water-soluble Vitamins in Moringa

Vitamin C

A superstar among stars, vitamin C (ascorbic acid) is one of the best studied substances supplied by the diet. This water-soluble vitamin is not a coenzyme but is rather required, among others, for the synthesis of collagen, a protein of the connective tissue in vertebrates. It does not sound too important but, in fact, without collagen our bodies would fall apart. One of the main symptoms of scurvy, stemming from lack of vitamin C, is the loss of teeth, but this is just the beginning of a painful, deadly disease. Scurvy is rare today but mild vitamin C deficiency is probably frequent. This is due to the fact that vitamin C is very sensitive and easily lost during cooking and processing of foods. Fresh fruits and greens have bioavailable vitamin C in various amounts. Juicing fruits and vegetables is also a great way of supplying vitamin C.

Since the human body is unable to manufacture vitamin C, we must acquire it from our diets - read: PLANTS.

Moringa contains abundant amounts of vitamin C. 100 g Moringa leaves contain more than 200 mg vitamin C, while 100 g orange juice has only about 40 mg of vitamin C. Moringa pods also contain twice the amount of vitamin C than oranges, per similar weight. As you know, citrus fruits (oranges, limes) are famous sources of vitamin C, until Moringa…

Vitamin C is surrounded by some controversy in terms of daily allowance and uses. All this fuss about vitamin C is due to its many other functions besides collagen formation. Some of the functions of vitamin C currently known are listed below:

- Supports and enhances the immune system in many ways, it has antiviral, antibacterial and anticancer properties.

- Supports the function and vitality of blood vessels. Therefore, it is beneficial in various conditions such as coronary disease (that affects the heart arteries), and may prevent strokes.

• Has powerful antioxidant capacity and antiaging properties. Vitamin C combats the oxidation of lipids, which has been linked to degeneration and premature aging, and works inside the cells to protect the genetic material from damage caused by free radicals. (Please review the chapter dedicated to antioxidants.)

• Supports detoxification and neutralization of toxins and pollutants by stimulating detoxifying enzymes.

It is clear now why so much interest and research has focused on this powerful vitamin which is even more beneficial to modern humans besieged by cancer, heart disease and countless pollutants such as environmental toxins.

While the recommended dose is only 60 mg of vitamin C per day (and that is found in just an ounce of Moringa leaves!), many argue for much higher needs at least 2 grams per day. But some claim that so much vitamin C is useless or even dangerous to our health.

Hmm...whom should I believe?

Most of the time I personally use the "BEAR method". Since our closest relatives in what concerns the digestive system, are omnivorous animals such as bears and monkeys (primates) who enjoy huge amounts of fresh greens and fruits loaded with vitamin C daily, we humans could also require huge amounts of vitamin C for proper health. In any case, 1-2 g of vitamin C cannot be dangerous to us - this is probably the amount of vitamin C that our ancestors ate during most of their long development as part of the animal kingdom, when they used to inhabit the wilderness and venerate trees.

There is a wealth of evidence about better health, reduced death rates from heart disease, cancer and other diseases, with 1-2 g of vitamin C per day for an adult. The more greens and fruits, the better. To enhance its antioxidant properties, it is best to supply vitamin C with other antioxidants, especially those found in plants, as there is strong evidence of synergy between various antioxidants. In other words, birds of a feather, work together. Since Moringa is also rich in various other antioxidants, it makes clear sense to consider it as an excellent source of bioavailable and efficient vitamin C.

The B Complex of Vitamins - to B or not to B...Healthy?

The following vitamins are part of a complex group of vital factors for our health. Their deficiency leads to serious diseases. Moringa is an excellent source of vitamins from the B complex group.

Vitamin B1

Vitamin B1, also known as thiamin, was the first B vitamin to be discovered. It is part of a large group of water-soluble vitamins, the B complex group. Vitamin B1 is vital for the production of energy within every cell and plays an essential role in the metabolism of various sugars (carbohydrates), which are a major source of energy. This vitamin is also needed for the processing of fats and proteins and for the normal function of the nervous system, heart and muscles.

For instance, vitamin B1 supports healthy development of the fat-like layer which surrounds most nerves (called the myelin sheath). In the absence of vitamin B1, this layer can degenerate or become damaged, therefore nervous transmission is problematic. Consequently, some of the symptoms of vitamin B deficiency are pain, prickly sensations and nerve deadening.

Interestingly, there is a decline in vitamin B1 levels with age, even in apparently healthy people. Serious deficiencies are not common in the Western world, although alcoholics, smokers, heavy drinkers of coffee and tea, people with malabsorption conditions (who cannot properly absorb nutrients) or poor eating habits may be deficient in this important vitamin. They might need 5-10 times the ordinary amount of vitamin B1!

Some might wonder what I mean by poor eating habits. Well, vitamin B1 is extremely unstable. From this point of view, poor eating habits that do not supply enough of the vitamin are actually very common. Examples of poor eating habits include:

- Eating mostly cooked, boiled or processed food such as decorticated grains.

- Eating processed grains like most breakfast cereals.

- Eating mostly white flour bakery products instead of whole grains.

- Long term refrigeration or freezing of foods where, after one year, more than 90 % of vitamin B1 in greens is lost and many other nutrients are also depleted.

If you think you share these habits (and many do!) you should consider introducing some rich, raw greens and vegetables in your diet. Pills wouldn't really help you as many supplements contain vitamin B1 in a biologically non-active form called thiamin hydrochloride.

What is the Vitamin B1 Amount I Should Take?

The recommended daily allowance for adults and children is between 1-2 mg per day. Now, you might think this is a small amount but vitamin B1 is not very abundant in foods, especially in our over-processed foods. As I said, it can easily vanish after cooking. For a list with vitamin B1 sources, see Table 5. Please note that Moringa leaves contain high amounts of vitamin B1 even compared with the best sources already known. The leaf powder is 10 times more concentrated in vitamin B1 than the leaves!

Table 5

Sources of Vitamin B1

Food (100 g)	Vitamin B1 (mg)
Asparagus (boiled)	0.12
Romaine lettuce	0.11
Tuna (broiled)	0.32
Green peas	0.20
Broccoli (raw)	0.03
Black beans (boiled)	0.20
Carrots (raw)	0.06
Corn (boiled)	0.18
Orange	0.11
Red meat (cooked)	0.15
Soy beans (cooked)	0.12
Moringa leaves	**0.21**
Moringa leaf powder	**2.6**

For those concerned about calories, keep in mind that tuna might have more vitamin B1 per weight, but provides many more calories than Moringa. Tuna also does not supply the broad spectrum of nutrients that Moringa provides.

Modern nutrition science has shown that vitamin B1 works hand in hand with vitamin B2 and vitamin B3, but Moringa "knew" this from the very beginning. As a wise plant, Moringa has decided to produce the other two vitamins as well, just to make it easier for us!

Vitamin B2

This vitamin is also known as riboflavin and is another vital factor required for the production of energy, proper use of oxygen and the metabolism of amino acids, fats and carbohydrates. Riboflavin is needed to activate vitamin B6 and assist the adrenal glands (that produce a variety of hormones regulating water and mineral balance). Riboflavin is important for red blood cell formation (these cells transport oxygen to the tissues), antibody production (antibodies protect us against infections) and growth. It is required for healthy mucus membranes, skin, for the absorption of iron and certain vitamins. And the list goes on…

What is the Daily Need of Vitamin B2?

The recommended dietary allowance (RDA) is about 1-1.5 mg per day, but some groups of people such as athletes, alcoholics and cancer patients, need more. The use of antibiotics and birth control pills also calls for more vitamin B2.

The good thing about this vitamin is that it is much more resistant to cooking, although it is sensitive to light. However, 70% of it is removed from whole wheat (a rich source) during processing of flour. This is another reason to replace white bread with whole grain bread.

So what is the content of vitamin B2 in Moringa? Moringa leaves compare with broccoli and spinach in B2 content, with about 0.07 mg per 100 g, while leaf powder has 20 mg per 100 g.

Vitamin B3

Vitamin B3 is the name given to nicotinamide and nicotinic acid. The disease "pellagra" is caused by a vitamin B3 deficiency. This vitamin is important for producing energy and the metabolism of proteins, fats and carbohydrates. Vitamin B3 also supports the digestive system function and promotes healthy skin and nerves. The body may produce vitamin B3 from the amino acid tryptophan, although a lot of tryptophan, 60 mg, is needed for 1 mg of vitamin B3.

Moringa leaves and pods contain 0.5-0.8 mg while the leaf powder has more than 8 mg vitamin B3 per 100 g.

Choline

Choline is part of several major phospholipids which are critical for normal membrane structure and cellular function. It is also used by the kidneys to maintain water balance and by the liver for synthesis of various compounds. Choline is used to produce the important neurotransmitter acetylcholine. Choline is particularly needed by athletes and people who exercise vigorously.

Choline is also vital for the developing fetus and the infant. It is important they receive adequate amounts of choline. Pregnancy and breast-feeding might deplete maternal stores of choline. Therefore, these conditions will also require extra choline.

Although the body can synthesize part of the choline in case of deficiency, it is recommended that humans intake enough choline from their diet. Diet recommendations call for about 400-550 mg/day for adults, proportionately, per body size.

Lipid Soluble Vitamins in Moringa

Vitamin A

Vitamin A is a lipid soluble vitamin of vital importance for vision, skin structure, and immune system functioning, among others. It is believed that this vitamin is the most important vitamin for immune protection against all kinds of infections and, possibly, cancer. It is the vitamin of HEALING and, without it, any recovery and healing process would be delayed or slowed. It is also known to be involved in bone development. Deficiency in vitamin A leads to disorders of the reproductive system, infections, xerophthalmia (a drying condition of the cornea of the eye), blindness and ultimately death. Vitamin A-related blindness in children was and still is a terrible medical situation in impoverished countries of the world.

Vitamin A is an excellent example to illustrate the power of a natural, balanced diet versus man-made vitamin pills. While vitamin A is essential for health, an excess of it can lead to serious medical problems, but an excess of vitamin A can only be achieved by abusing vitamin A supplements. Since it is a liposoluble vitamin, it can accumulate in the body (liver) and lead to toxicity. (Water-soluble vitamins like the C and B complex are eliminated easier when in excess.)

I know that Eskimos are going to contradict me here: one can achieve excess of naturally-occurring vitamin A not only with pills but also by eating polar bear liver! Did you know that you should never eat polar bear liver? The vitamin A found in a modest piece of polar bear liver is more than a two years supply for a human. Okay, as long as you do not hunt the poor polar bear for your vitamin A supply, you need not worry about an excess of vitamin A from food. But you should worry about having ENOUGH vitamin A in your food.

Here comes Moringa.

Moringa contains extremely rich amounts of vitamin A in its plant form - provitamin A or beta-carotene. Beta-carotene is the molecule that gives carrots their orange color. It is a member of the carotenoid family. Carotenoids are an important group of natural pigments responsible for many of the yellow and orange colors of fruit and vegetables, as well as the wonderful color of the fall leaves.

Beta-carotene and vitamin A are very closely related in structure. The body produces vitamin A from beta-carotene, and if the beta-carotene is in excessive quantities, it can be eliminated or deposited in the fat tissue - thus no toxicity results from ingesting large amounts of plants containing provitamin A as beta-carotene. Beta-carotene is a safe source of vitamin A. Interestingly, carotenes from natural sources are absorbed 4 to 10 times better than synthetic carotenes, such as those found in most vitamin pills, tablets or capsules. I emphasize again, plants are the best, safest source of vitamins, and vitamin A is one of the best examples.

But even from natural sources, only one-third of the beta-carotene is absorbed and only one-half of what is absorbed is converted to vitamin A. Why is this important? Because you have to search for the best, richest sources of carotene possibly existent to be sure you obtain enough vitamin A. One of the best sources is Moringa leaves. Moringa leaves contain almost 7-8 mg of beta-carotene, while the leaf powder has twice that amount in 100 g. Your daily needs are about 1 mg but some have suggested more, especially for protection against ultraviolet radiation from excessive exposure to the sun. Natural beta-carotene also guards against heart disease and can keep harmful lipoproteins containing cholesterol from damaging the heart and coronary arteries and prevents certain types of cancers, and stroke.

I am sure you are anxious to know how Moringa's beta-carotene content compares with other plant foods. Besides animal foods, such as whole milk, butter, egg yolk and liver, the best sources of vitamin A as carotene are green leafy vegetables and colorful fruits and roots such as mangoes and carrots. You will be surprised to find that Moringa leaves have more beta-carotene than the carrot, famous precisely for its content of beta-carotene! For a reality check, please consult Table 6.

Table 6

Beta-Carotene Content and Corresponding Vitamin A Equivalents in Various Foods*

Food	Beta-Carotene mg/100g	Vitamin A equivalent mg/100g
Coriander leaves	7,000—8,000	1,166—1,300
Cabbage	1,300	218
Spinach	3,600	600
Carrot	1,300—2,600	215—430
Mango	3,000	500
Orange	200	35
Pumpkin	650 -700	100—120
Moringa leaves	**7,000—8,000**	**1,166—1,300**

*Animals do not produce beta-carotene

Another important reason to supply plenty of beta-carotene is its powerful antioxidant capacity, a property not related to vitamin A. The chapter "Antioxidants in Moringa" will describe in detail the harmful effects of oxidants and how they can be annihilated by antioxidants found abundantly in plants.

Beta-carotene blocks the action of activated oxygen molecules or "free radicals" that contribute to aging and can damage all cells. Beta-carotene also enhances the activities of natural killer cells (a type of blood cell with a suggestive name) and other cells of the immune system that protect the body against infections and cancer. It has been clearly proven that beta-carotene may prevent cancers of the epithelial cells that make up the outer layer of skin, mouth, lungs, stomach, intestines, bladder and glands in the breasts. In some cases it even reverses precancerous conditions! Beta-carotene in man-made supplements has not demonstrated cancer-protective properties, on contrary. The reasons for this may be multiple or it may be that scientists do not yet understand them. It is possible that, in order to perform its protective function in cancer, beta-carotene needs other substances that are found in natural sources (very complex by nature), but not in the man-made versions.

IMPORTANT: to provide the best anti-cancer activity, beta-carotene should be mixed with the vitamins C and E, and selenium. Moringa has them all.

Vitamin E

This vitamin is also known as tocopherol, and is an essential fat-soluble factor. It has a broad role in promoting health, from enhancing fertility and energy production, to preventing aging, heart disease and cancer.

The main benefit of vitamin E is that it is a powerful antioxidant. It protects cells from oxidation by neutralizing unstable free radicals which cause cell damage. Vitamin E gives up one of its electrons to the electron deficient free radicals, making them more stable, thus less dangerous. While vitamin E acts as a donor, it also protects other antioxidants (like vitamin A) from being oxidized, therefore prolonging their effectiveness. This is another fine example of how compounds cooperate inside of our bodies and why it is important to offer ourselves a rich, complex diet from natural sources! We will discuss again antioxidants and vitamin E in the exciting chapter "Antioxidants in Moringa".

The antioxidant ability of vitamin E (similarly to other antioxidants) contributes to prevent premature aging, degenerative diseases - including heart disease, arthritis, diabetes and cancer. It also protects the body from pollution, increases stamina and reduces or prevents hot flashes in menopause. Vitamin E is also used externally, in various creams for skin treatments, promoting young-looking skin, healing and reducing scar tissue from forming.

What is the daily recommended dose and how can Moringa contribute? Adults should ingest at least 10 mg per day of vitamin E (together with a wide range of antioxidants like vitamin C and beta-carotene). If your diet includes plenty of refined carbohydrates and fried foods, if you are on birth control pills or hormone replacement therapy, if you are exposed to pollution (who isn't?), then more vitamin E might be needed. A good source of vitamin E should provide at least 10 % of the daily needs, with relatively few calories. Remember, vitamin E is generally found in fatty foods (rich in calories), being liposoluble by nature. Moringa contains large amounts of vitamin E in the leaves (very few calories) and in the leaf powder - about 110 mg per 100 g of leaf powder or 100 g of oil. In addition, Moringa also contains antioxidants such as vitamin C, beta-carotene and others - just a great mix!

SUMMARY

Vitamins are absolutely essential for growth and maintenance of a healthy life.

Most vitamins are not produced by our bodies, therefore they must be supplied by the diet.

Moringa is rich in many vitamins, particularly in Vitamin C, proVitamin A (beta-carotene) Vitamins B1 and E. These abundant vitamins in Moringa exceed those commonly found in most other plants.

Many of the vitamins in Moringa have powerful antioxidant and antiaging properties.

A healthful diet, including plenty of fruits and vegetables is the best and safest source of vitamins.

"Verde que te quiero verde. Verde viento.
Verde ramas."

"Green I love you green.
Green Wind.
Green branches."

Federico Garcia Lorca

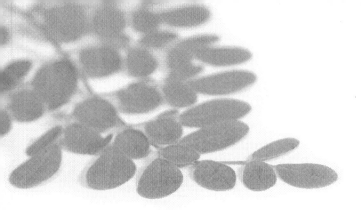

CHLOROPHYLL

C hlorophyll is one of the most beloved painted and sung colors of all. Chlorophyll, nature's green is all you! Pigment and medicine, complex chemical and source of energy, chlorophyll still fascinates scientists. No wonder, this green pigment of plants (which incorporates magnesium in its molecule) is involved in the most important biochemical reaction on earth, photosynthesis. Our lives could not be possible without it. Chlorophyll is the master chemical at the base of all of our food supply and oxygen production.

Throughout history, healing has been associated with green. We feel better and relaxed when we see green, probably because we, like all other animals, have been living with plants since our beginnings. Maybe green means "home" for our souls.

Green plants like Moringa are loaded with precious chlorophyll. And, although no daily allowance was ever established for it and no one calls it an essential vitamin, chlorophyll presence in the diet could be very beneficial for your health. The reasons are multiple, although not everybody agrees on them (just like for vitamin C and so many others…). But let's first introduce our subject.

Chlorophyll, often referred to as "the blood of plants", is closely related to hemoglobin - the red pigment of red blood cells responsible for oxygen transport in many animals. The main difference between the two molecules is the metallic element in the center. In human blood, hemoglobin consists of iron, while in chlorophyll, the metallic element is magnesium. Some believe that this resemblance helps the chlorophyll to be better absorbed and used to "build-up" blood and fight anemia. Some scientists and nutritionists do not believe it is absorbed internally (to reach the blood) but rather that it may act locally to support the health of the mouth, stomach and intestinal tract.

In either case, there is much evidence that chlorophyll could cure or ease acute infections of the respiratory tract and sinuses, chronic ulcers, and bad breath; it also accelerates wound healing and has been shown in animal studies to nullify the cancer-inducing effects of a variety of environmental (including food!) toxins. Other studies have shown that chlorophyll supports liver function and detoxification of the body. It sounds very much like other plant pigments - please review the beta-carotene and carotenoids. It is reasonable to believe that this green pigment acts like other plant pigments (such as carotenoids) and is beneficial to our health. In fact, I always felt better and more energetic when I ate green, for whatever reason, so I make sure I keep chlorophyll present in a natural form in my diet. Learned from my omnivorous cousins, the bear and monkey.

Moringa is one of the very few foods that contain chlorophyll together with so many other nutrients (vitamins, minerals, proteins, beneficial fats), and has a great taste. Dark-green vegetables and herbs like Romaine lettuce, spinach or parsley are excellent sources of chlorophyll, but they do not provide many of the other nutrients of Moringa.

*"The true meaning of life is to plant trees,
under whose shade you do not expect to sit."*

Nelson Henderson

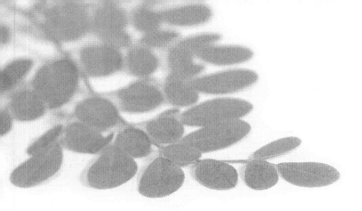

BETA-SITOSTEROL IN MORINGA

Sterol Against Sterol

Hold on, this is not a scene from "Invasion of the Body Snatchers", but rather a real biological "warfare" between two similar substances of the sterol family: beta-sitosterol and cholesterol. A sterol is a complex chemical related to steroid hormones but which also relates to alcohols. The sterols are naturally occurring substances in plants and animals and have many functions.

Cholesterol is mainly found in animals. It plays essential roles in the formation of cell membranes, synthesis of hormones and vitamin D, therefore its presence is vital for health. Too high levels in the blood (actually in the serum) are dangerous, though. High cholesterol levels are a main risk factor for cardiovascular disease. Beta-sitosterol is a specific plant sterol, from the family of phytosterols. As mentioned before, it has a chemical structure that is very similar to cholesterol - the much maligned serum fat that we all try to keep under control.

Beta-sitosterol has been shown to reduce blood cholesterol levels! This is due to their competition for absorption in the intestines: since the two sterols are similar, beta-sitosterol "tricks" the intestines and inhibits the absorption of food cholesterol. In other words, although beta-sitosterol is not well absorbed by the body, when consumed with animal fat cholesterol, it efficiently blocks cholesterol absorption. Consequently, lower serum cholesterol levels can result. Beta-sitosterol also improves other blood lipids besides cholesterol levels, and brings them to a more normal range.

Here you have it - maybe you could enjoy your steak WITH Moringa after all! Maybe, but don't take this to an excess of steak, of course. Remember, the liver itself also produces cholesterol. (Please review "Fats in Moringa" for facts on fats and how Moringa's oleic acid can help.)

Moringa is very rich in beta-sitosterol and related substances, and this is another excellent reason to include it in your diet. If you remember from the chapter on fats, Moringa contains another factor against high cholesterol - oleic acid. In any case, you might need extra beta-sitosterol. It is believed that the average American diet lacks this component, since it generally includes few veggies.

~ Plant sterols like beta-sitosterol are also proven to be very beneficial in preventing and treating prostate problems like prostate enlargement due to aging. Plant sterols improve many of the prostate-related symptoms. Even more, beta-sitosterol acts against some forms of cancer. It has been found to reduce the growth of prostate and colon cancer cells.

Among other medical benefits of beta-sitosterol:

- It boosts the immune defense.

- It has anti-inflammatory properties.

- It helps normalize the blood sugar and supports the pancreas (which produces insulin - the hormone controlling blood sugar).

- It helps to heal ulcers.

- It can alleviate cramps.

The list could go on, but I think you get the idea ~ -Moringa has many weapons against high cholesterol and its potential harmful effects.

"He who plants a tree, plants a hope."

Lucy Larcou - "Plant a Tree"

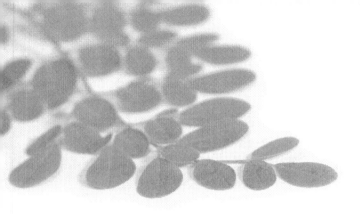

PLANT HORMONES

Zeatin - a Powerful Antiagine Factor

By now, you must be impressed by the richness and versatility of this incredible tree. Everywhere it grows, in India or Niger, Arabic countries or Nicaragua, Moringa has been embraced and recognized as a valuable nutritive and healing source. In regions with harsh climates, where food resources are scarce, just 25 grams of Moringa leaf powder can provide a child with about half the protein amount, all the calcium and vitamin A, a quarter of vitamin C and three quarters of iron needed daily! What a nutritious power plant, indeed. Recent studies have discovered that Moringa might have even more exciting properties than previously thought. Biochemical analysis has revealed that the Moringa leaves and leaf powder contain unusually large amounts of plant hormones named cytokinins, such as zeatin and the related dihydrozeatin.

Cytokinins function as plant hormones, which are naturally occurring growth promoters and factors that delay senescence (the process of aging) in many plants. Furthermore, research studies have shown that plant cytokinins may be very active in animals, as well. We will discuss below the functions and significance of cytokinins, in general and zeatin in particular, in the process of aging. You will be surprised to find out how zeatin can help your skin, hair and more. Remember when I called Moringa a beautician? If you were wondering then, now zeatin should solve this puzzle...in a beautiful way.

Cytokinins are compounds with a structure resembling adenine - one of the major components of the genetic material encoding information in the cell nucleus. Cytokinins have been found in almost all higher plants, as well as simpler organisms such as fungi and bacteria (single cell organisms), therefore they must play a vital role in the lives of plants. Indeed, cytokinins regulate a wide number of processes such as:

- flowering.

- germination of seeds.

- healing of wounds.

- the accumulation and synthesis of nutrients (proteins, minerals).

- ultimately, cytokinins control plant growth by stimulating the cell division (known as cytokinesis) and multiplication of plant parts. They stimulate the synthesis of nucleic acids (which encode the genetic information necessary for cell functioning and multiplication) and proteins.

In other words, thanks to the dynamic cytokinins, plants know when to grow more leaves or when to expand their roots, when to sit silenced, or when they should bloom again. One could compare a cytokinin with the director of a huge philharmonic orchestra of cells. The director gives the entry for every cell type, I mean the start for division and growth, or signals their end. All has to be, of course, harmonious and perfectly in tune with Nature's music (seasons, light, temperature, humidity), otherwise plants would not survive.

In addition, cytokinins delay the aging, the destruction of plant tissues and postpone death. In the 1930s, it was discovered that tomato roots could be cultured in an artificial medium indefinitely, while continuing to grow roots, if they were supplied a natural plant extract containing (what proved later to be) cytokinins. Since then, scientists have uncovered many of the miraculous plant hormones and today there are more than 200 known natural and synthetic cytokinins.

Kinetin was the first cytokinin discovered, although it is not sure if plants synthesize it, therefore it is considered a synthetic cytokinin. The most common and the most active naturally occurring cytokinin in plants is zeatin, which was first isolated from corn (named *Zea mays* in Latin). Let's explore now how zeatin can delay aging.

Cytokinins and Aging

How do cytokinins delay aging in plants? What about their effects on animals and humans? These questions are not yet fully answered, although new and exciting data reveals insights about their mechanism of action in plants and animals.

Briefly, cytokinins may act through a number of ways to stimulate the enzymes and processes involved in regeneration of tissues, while protecting against degrading enzymes and damaging free radicals. (Enzymes are the workforce of the body; substances that activate or inactivate all physiological processes. However, some enzymes are involved in destroying and possibly damaging cellular structures.) In order to understand the effects of zeatin and other cytokinins, we should first review some of the key issues about aging in plants and animals.

Organism aging is characterized by a declining ability to respond to stress, increased biochemical imbalances and the occurrence of diseases (especially degenerative diseases), with death as the ultimate consequence. While we tend to notice mostly the external effects of aging, for instance on skin and visual acuity, actually aging occurs first at the level of the minuscule living units - the cells. Every day, cells age and die in our bodies, and in plants for that matter. Cellular senescence (aging) can be demonstrated in the laboratory: various isolated cells have a limited ability to divide in culture. In other words, they divide and grow for a fixed number of times, and then they stop multiplying and die. A variety of cell biology alterations occurs as the cells progress from young and vigorous, to old and dry. As a consequence, we all function according to a biological clock, ultimately dictated by our cells. Genetic and environmental factors may affect the life span of cells and organisms, as a whole.

Importantly, it is believed that certain nutrients may affect the rate and occurrence of aging. This gives much hope to many that human aging can be slowed and has spurred intense research efforts within the field of senescence.

Surely enough, we all hope for a long and healthy life, but how to reach that is still under debate. Groucho Marx once said that anyone can get old; we just have to live long enough! Longevity requires that we nourish our bodies properly, support the extraordinary healing power within us and fight diseases wisely - by using natural laws and the best medicines. A wholesome diet that strengthens our inner powers and delays aging should include the necessary nutrients, plenty of vitamins, essential microelements and protective phytochemicals that minimize tissue damage inherently occurring with age. Among the phytochemicals, cytokinins might play a crucial role.

Various experiments have shown that cytokinins like zeatin or kinetin have potent antiaging and protective effects in animals (including humans), similar to their activity in plants. Could that be possible, taking into consideration the physiological and anatomical differences between plant and animal kingdoms?

Well, it seems so. Plants, like animals, do have regulated growth, determined phases of tissue differentiation, specialized cell types and sophisticated communication between cells. Apart from obvious differences, plants and animals share a majority of biological compounds (proteins, lipids, sugars, vitamins, and minerals), and their genetic material encodes information according to similar formulas. Even basic cell organization is quite similar, as well. Plant cytokinins might be physiologically compared to animal hormones -endogenous substances that control development, growth, metabolism and other various functions in animals.

Zeatin, similar to kinetin and other cytokinins, has potent antioxidant properties as well. As described in the chapter dedicated to the antioxidants, aging can be equated to an increased oxidation of cell components such as proteins, genetic material and lipids. Upon oxidation, they change or lose their normal functions, thus leading to a disruption of normal physiological processes. Plants are the main source of powerful antioxidant substances that can trap and neutralize the damaging free oxygen radicals. By acting as an antioxidant, zeatin becomes another valuable substance in the fight against premature aging.

Evidence for the antiaging effects of zeatin and other cytokinins is presented below. We have seen that cells in plants and animals divide for a preset number of times, then they stop dividing and die. This process dictates organism aging, and is controlled, at its turn, by a number of factors - both internal and external to the plant or animal. We have also described briefly that oxidation of vital cellular components triggers aging, often prematurely. Plants are considered today as the main source of powerful antioxidant and antiaging substances. Therefore humans should include a broad variety of plants, including fruits, herbs, legumes, roots, and others, in their daily diet, in order to delay aging and maintain excellent health.

Scientists, in their quest for understanding life and improving its quality, have gone one step further and purified certain plant components. These were studied in the laboratory or field and applied to various experimental systems in order to elucidate their mechanism of action. Upon careful consideration, the most active plant components were selected, concentrated, purified, and many can be found on the market as supplements for human diet. Since cytokinins have proved to be such an exciting group of phytochemicals, scientists have put them to the test.

- **Cytokinins have proven to delay biochemical modifications associated with aging in cultured human cells.** Experiments conducted in Denmark, in association with American researchers, have shown that kinetin solutions that are applied to human cells (fibroblasts) lead to significant delays in the onset of aging and cell death. The treated cells maintained much longer their youthful characteristics (biochemical composition, skeletal and shape organization, active protein and genetic material synthesis). They were not accumulating age-pigment like substances. These effects are seen as preventative, since no additional cell divisions were triggered.
  - Human cells were growing continuously and remained younger while under the influence of kinetin.

- **Zeatin protects the skin.** Zeatin has demonstrated even better properties than kinetin in a similar experimental system. Human skin cells treated with zeatin retain their functions longer, do not accumulate biochemical damage associated with aging and are more resistant to environmental stresses. Besides its mechanism on cell growth, and as described above, zeatin has potent antioxidant properties. It can increase the activity of known antioxidant enzymes, such as catalases, that naturally fight aging and free oxygen radicals. In other words, zeatin acts synergistically with other inner antiaging molecules, orchestrating a stronger offensive against senescence.

These impressive results have lead to the development of skin and hair care products containing kinetin and zeatin, in Europe and the USA. These effective and unique preparations protect against environmental damage, delay skin aging and improve skin barrier functions (allowing better humidity retention and elasticity). By comparison with other antiaging substances, cytokinins do NOT induce peeling, dryness or exfoliation with consequent thinning of the skin. In other words, youthful skin without risks! The effectiveness in maintaining normal cell functions and safety for local use could make cytokinins the ingredients of choice for preserving healthy skin. Another conclusion to be drawn from here is that cytokinins work in living animal organisms, not only in their cultured, isolated cells.

Clinical studies with human subjects on cytokinins treatment have also demonstrated an excellent efficacy in photo damaged skin (visible light and UV damage). These preparations reduced skin wrinkles and roughness within 8-24 weeks in almost all patients treated. Scientists are further testing and proposing the introduction of cytokinin combinations for even better activity.

- **Zeatin protects animals against neuronal toxicity induced by age-specific proteins.** One of the main characteristics of brain aging is the accumulation of modified, non-functional proteins that often aggregate as insoluble particles. These are named amyloids and are believed to play an essential role in the development of brain degenerative diseases such as dementia. Since people are living longer and the number of cases of dementia has increased dramatically, scientists are intensively looking for preventative treatments against age-re-lated brain diseases. Studies have shown that zeatin administered to mice can effectively protect them against memory and brain performance loss triggered by amyloids and chemical agents. It makes sense to believe that, if zeatin is an antioxidant and stimulates proper skin cell functioning and metabolism, it could also work as an antioxidant and protector for the neurons (the brain's main cells). Further studies are ongoing to clarify the importance of zeatin supplements for delaying brain aging.

Zeatin has another interesting property that could be exploited in the treatment of some forms of dementia (Alzheimer's disease). This cytokinin can enhance neuronal function and transmission of the signals by increasing the amounts of acetylcholine (a natural substance used by neurons for signaling from one to another). In Alzheimer's disease, acetylcholine concentration is much lower than normal; therefore the transmission of information by neurons becomes defective and slow. Zeatin is one of the most powerful substances that increases the amount of acetylcholine in the brain by inhibiting its degradation by specific enzymes. In summary, zeatin was proven to exhibit antioxidant, neuroprotective effects through a number of different mechanisms. Its presence could be very beneficial against brain senescence.

• Zeatin and cancer. One of the most frequent diseases of old age is cancer. Actually "cancer" is a complex set of many diseases, all characterized by some common biochemical changes occurring in cancerous (tumor) cells. Cell oxidation plays a major role in cancer development. Due to accumulated defects in the genetic material, cells lose the tight growth and function control that keeps them healthy and "well-behaved". The cancerous cells start to divide too rapidly and many become nonfunctional, leading to tumors. Many of the tumor cells behave as "non-differentiated". The cells are unable to decide which type of structure and growth path to take.

It was shown that zeatin can inhibit cancer cell growth by "directing" them on the right path, and differentiating them into normal cells. The normal cells thus reverted, regain the normal, tight control that keeps them from dividing chaotically. These studies on zeatin's effects in cancer are still ongoing, but they show great promise.

But what is the concentration of zeatin in Moringa? Is Moringa a common source of zeatin or rather an exceptional one?

Zeatin is found in many, if not most, superior plants. The amount of zeatin in various plants or even the same plant may vary according to the phase of growth, season, temperature, part of the plant analyzed, the use of fertilizers, etc. Scientists have found zeatin in very low concentration in plants. (Generally, plant hormones are very active substances; therefore their concentration does not need to be high.) Of course, many plants have not been tested yet for zeatin concentrations, but for those tested, the zeatin amounts vary between .00002 mcg/g material to .02 mcg/g. The zeatin concentration in Moringa leaves gathered from various parts of the world was found to be very high, between 5 mcg and 200mcg/g material, or thousands of times more concentrated than in most plants studied so far. [IBC Laboratory, Tucson, AZ] We do not yet know what is the significance of this unusually high amount of zeatin: maybe it could be linked to the very fast growth of this plant, or to its extraordinary nutritive richness, or to both. Definitely, it is not just a coincidence. Moringa is so unusual in so many ways. We do not yet know how zeatin is absorbed in the body from Moringa, or how and if it affects the internal tissues. But, as detailed above, in cell cultures and human skin, zeatin is very beneficial and can prevent or reduce damage due to environmental factors. We are anxiously waiting for more studies to explain the "zeatin effect", and believe it could be as spectacular from inside as from outside of the body (or external application, as performed in the studies).

SUMMARY

Zeatin is a normal, dynamic hormone in many plants. It functions to control growth, healing and the accumulation of nutrients.

Zeatin delays aging by its influence on cell division and antioxidant properties.

Recent and ongoing studies have shown that zeatin and related plant hormones have antiaging, skin-protective and antioxidant properties in animals, including humans.

Zeatin protects animals against neuronal toxicity induced by age-specific factors.

Zeatin inhibits cancer cells (in laboratory setting) and induces their differentiation into normal cells.

Moringa is indeed extraordinarily rich in zeatin.

"The most beautiful thing we can experience is the mysterious. It is the source of all true art and science. Something deeply hidden had to be behind things. There are two ways in which to view our existence: a world without any miracles and a world that is nothing but miracles; I chose the latter."

Albert Einstein

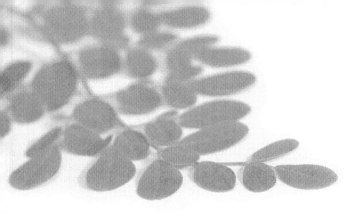

ANTIOXIDANTS IN MORINGA

Are you ready for a complex and exciting subject? If not, take a break and have a green tea which is teaming with antioxidants. After you refresh yourself, come back, find a comfortable seat and let's start.

So far we have described a number of essential, vital nutrients for normal physiology. We just can't be healthy without them in the long run. Maybe your head is spinning with data, but don't worry, you will learn what is necessary with time. This is the last chapter dedicated to another extremely important group of naturally occurring substances in Moringa and in some other plants - the antioxidants. There is a tremendous amount of information and scientific data about antioxidants; you can find magazines and books dealing specifically with them. My purpose here is to give you a short but comprehensive introduction to some of the antioxidants found so far in Moringa. I say "so far" since Moringa has just recently been studied by scientists. We may expect many pleasant surprises and beneficial health discoveries as this wonderful plant becomes better known.

- According to our present knowledge, Moringa contains specific plant pigments with demonstrated potent antioxidant properties such as the carotenoids - lutein, alpha-carotene and beta-carotene, xanthins, chlorophyll and others.

- Moringa contains powerful antioxidant vitamins such as vitamin C, E and A (pro-vitamin A as beta-carotene).

- Moringa has essential micronutrients with antioxidant activity or directly linked to this process: selenium and zinc.

- Moringa (leaves, seeds, pods) contains other phytochemicals with known powerful antioxidant ability such as kaempferol, quercetin, rutin and caffeoylquinic acids.

Some of these substances were already covered and their mechanism of action was briefly described (vitamins A, C, E, selenium, zinc, and chlorophyll), so I will focus on the new substances such as quercetin, lutein and the others. But let me first explain in a few words what tissue oxidation really means and why it is so important to reduce its consequences at cellular level.

What is "Oxidation" or "Oxidative Stress"?

Just by living, eating and breathing, our bodies produce free radicals every second, such as single oxygen molecules, superoxide radicals, nitric oxide and other unstable oxygen and nitrogen containing molecules. Oxygen is vital for living on earth, it is present in every cell, participates in every chemical reaction in the cells, one way or another, but its chemical combinations can be very unstable. These unstable, "restless" chemicals are missing electrons, and therefore are in constant search for other molecules that might provide them with the needed electrons. Remember from chemistry class, any atom is stable (less or non-reactive) when its electrons (negativelycharged particles) are paired. Electrons don't enjoy loneliness. Free radicals steal electrons from other molecules (proteins, lipids, genetic material, others) in the cells, and, in this process, they create other unstable molecules, creating a vicious circle. This unauthorized, ferocious theft of electrons is named oxidation. Oxidation of substances can be equated to damage and aging. Oxidative stress is caused by an excess of reactive radicals, which our defense mechanisms can no longer remove.

Any cell in our body is subjected to the threat and damage of oxidation constantly. It is estimated that a human cell generates billions of free radicals per day. Of course, our cells don't just sit there and wait to be bombarded and destroyed; no, they have developed powerful methods of counterattack - the antioxidants. Antioxidants occur naturally in plants and animals, and they can belong to various chemical classes, as we have seen. They can be vitamins, enzymes, metals, or other chemical families. Without them, oxidation will quickly lead to irreversible damage and death of cells and tissues.

Free radicals or oxidants (electron thieves) attack all cells, work against our various tissues, impact the immune system (our guardian against infections and cancer) and play a major role in the development of all chronic degenerative diseases (atherosclerosis, Alzheimer's disease). Oxidation at the level of genetic material - that encodes all the information required for normal function and replacement of "used" substances - leads to mutations, or changes in the encoded information, and the appearance of aberrant substances. It is believed that this is one of the mechanisms leading to cancer.

How Can Antioxidants Protect Against Oxidation?

Antioxidants donate electrons.

For instance, phytochemicals can donate an electron, accompanied by a hydrogen atom, from their hydroxyl (OH) groups, to a free radical. This electron stabilizes and inactivates the damaging radical; it pairs its ex-lonely electron. In the process, the phytochemical becomes an "aroxyl" radical which is considerably more stable than the free radical it has annihilated. In other words, the antioxidant becomes a sort of radical but of a non-dangerous type. The overall result is the interruption of damaging oxidative chain reaction. The more hydroxyl groups (OH) an antioxidant has, the more powerful it is.

Now you can introduce the antioxidants, and ask for their protection in your prayers; they might be your best friends. It is clear, I hope, why it is so important to provide daily vitamins, minerals, beneficial nutrients (proteins, essential fatty acids) and antioxidants (plant-derived chemicals mostly). Antioxidants are not only for replacement of the lost or "consumed" nutrients or build-up of the body and the support of new cells, but, very importantly, for supporting the fight against aging and damaging of each and every cell. No matter what diet suits you best or what you prefer to eat, or how many calories you consume, antioxidants have to be present in your diet if you love life.

SUMMARY

Normal biochemical reactions inside our bodies create unstable molecules = free radicals.

Free radicals steal electrons from other molecules, in this process damaging them and creating new free radicals.

- Every day, every cell is hit by numerous free radicals.

- Antioxidants donate electrons to the electron-starved free radicals, thus rendering them tame and stable.

The more antioxidants in our bodies, the less cellular damage and diseases.

Antioxidants work better in complex combinations with other antioxidants.

Plants are the main and richest source of antioxidants for humans.

Moringa's antioxidants belong to various chemical classes, and research has shown that combinations of such compounds are very effective and powerful in neutralizing free radicals. Vitamin C works best in the presence of beta-carotene and selenium. Vitamin C (which is very rich in Moringa) also supports the antioxidant activity of polyphenols (compounds with many hydroxyl - OH - groups) such as the antioxidants quercetin or kaempferol, also found in Moringa leaves.

Without being overly complicated, let's take a closer look at the other important antioxidants in Moringa, not previously covered.

Alpha-carotene, a carotenoid related to beta -carotene, is another powerful antioxidant. Carotenoids are fat-soluble pigments that prevent oxidation in plant cells and act similarly in animals. This carotene can also be used by the body to produce vitamin A and it is believed that alpha-carotene may be more powerful than beta-carotene in inhibiting cancer (tumor) growth. All dietary carotenoids are thought to be very beneficial by decreasing the risk of diseases, particularly cardiovascular ones, certain cancers and eye disease. Carotenoids enhance natural immunity and protect against infections and cancers. Other carotenoids that have been the most studied for these effects are lutein and zeaxanthin. Both are found in Moringa leaves.

Lutein, another beneficial plant pigment, is especially recognized for its protective eye and skin effects. It is found in dark green leafy vegetables.

Moringa has extraordinary amounts of lutein! 100 g of leaves contain more than 70 mg, while the recommended daily amount for the best protective antioxidant activity is 5-20 mg for an adult. The more lutein, the better. Lutein promotes healthy eyes by reducing the risk of macular degeneration (irreversible damage of the retina, thus leading to blindness). As an antioxidant, it appears to reduce harmful free radicals, and it also filters the high-energy, blue wavelengths of visible light. Blue light (from indoor lighting and sunlight) is believed to induce oxidative stress in human organs exposed to light, such as the eyes and skin. (Blue light is not an ultraviolet light of the invisible spectrum. Ultraviolet light is also dangerous for the eyes, though.) It is believed that most Americans do not get enough lutein in their diets. Eat your greens!

Zeaxanthin is another carotenoid beneficial for the eyes, found in Moringa leaves. Scientists have established that zeaxanthin plays essential roles in protecting the retina of the eye from the negative effects of light. How can that be? The retina has a particular affinity for two carotenoids of the hundreds possibly present in a (healthy) diet, lutein and zeaxanthin. The retina selectively accumulates these two; therefore their concentration is very high in the retina, specifically in the part known as "macula", which is responsible for visual acuity.

Since lutein and zeaxanthin absorb blue light, and because they are powerful antioxidants, it is hypothesized that they protect the retina. Indeed, these two related carotenoids, lutein and zeaxanthin, are your best allies in the fight against macular degeneration - the most prevalent cause of vision loss in the elderly. More than 17 million Americans have symptoms of macular degeneration and about 2 million have functional blindness, while 500,000 new cases are diagnosed each year.

With the greatest due respect for carotenoids of all colors and sources, I would like to end their description by saying:

- Long-term inadequate intake of carotenoids is associated with chronic diseases such as heart disease, cancers, and blindness.

- Carotenoids are fat-soluble substances and, as such, require the presence of dietary fat for proper absorption! Another reason to make sure you eat your good fats.

- If you smoke cigarettes or drink alcohol, you may have lower than normal blood levels of carotenoids (cigarette smoke destroys carotenoids).

Other antioxidants in Moringa include kaempferol, quercetin, rutin and caffeoylquinic acids.

Quercetin, rutin and kaempferol are three related flavonoids (a type of phytochemicals) with powerful antioxidant properties found in certain plants. Moringa is very rich in these extremely active flavonoids. Their chemical structure is quite complicated and so are the details about doses and concentrations in various plants. But let's remain at the most important issue for us, and that is health benefits. These flavonoids have been thoroughly researched for their anti-inflam-matory, anti-allergic, antiatherosclerotic, anti-asthmatic and anticancer properties.

Quercetin inhibits the production and release of histamine and other allergic and inflammatory substances. Histamine is a substance that contributes to allergy symptoms such as runny nose, watery eyes and swelling of soft tissue including the face. In laboratory and animal studies, quercetin and related flavonoids have anti-inflammatory properties; for example, quercetin inhibits the type of inflammation that occurs in the joints of those with arthritis.

Quercetin studies suggest that it decreases pain and other symptoms in men with chronic prostatitis (inflammation of the prostate) while laboratory studies have shown that quercetin may inhibit the growth of prostate cancer cells. Research continues as quercetin and related flavonoids have been shown in animal studies to inhibit the growth of cancer cells, including those from colon, breast and lung tumors. Most of these effects are due to the antioxidant properties, although these flavonoids might have specific effects on various tissues.

Rutin and quercetin work together, that is they complement each other, and should be taken together. In Moringa you have them together. One of the major benefits of rutin is strengthening of the blood capillaries (the finest vessels). Scientists believe that quercetin and rutin work together in improving capillary fragility and arterial elasticity and, therefore, may help those who bruise or bleed easily. Other quercetin and rutin synergistic activities include:

- stimulation of the elimination of cholesterol from the body.

- supporting the body to utilize vitamin C, another powerful antioxidant.

- maintaining of the protein collagen - which is what keeps the skin healthy, elastic and firm (the breakdown of collagen is what leads to wrinkles).

Caffeoylquinic acids belong to a family of very well studied antioxidants with incredible healing properties. The main plant known to contain such compounds and where most of the research was done is the artichoke (*Cynara* in

Latin). *Cynara* is famous precisely for its content of caffeoylquinic acids and related compounds which give it its hepatoprotector qualities. Cynara is present in multiple formulations around the world today, although it has been used since Roman times for the treatment and support of the liver and gallbladder. The Germans have thoroughly studied this miraculous plant and use it in various ailments of the gastro-intestinal system, in children, adults and elderly. Around the world, *Cynara* extract is often standardized to contain 1-2 % of caffeoylquinic acids. Moringa leaves contain 0.5-1 % caffeoylquinic acids, coming very close to the content that makes *Cynara* famous!

What benefits do caffeoylquinic acids really bring? They are considered choleretic (bile increasing; bile is vital for the digestion of dietary fats), hepatoprotective (therefore effective against hepatitis and other liver diseases), cholesterol-reducing, and diuretic. As you know, the liver is our chemical factory that digests food, produces energy, and detoxifies the body, to mention just a few of its main functions. The liver is the only organ that can regenerate itself if parts of it are removed, similar to the famous lizard's tail. Whenever the liver is sick, there is a total depletion of energy and vitality - those who have experienced hepatitis (inflammation and infection of the liver) can tell you about the terrifying feeling of total weakness.

Caffeoylquinic acids (naturally occurring in plants) have been studied in clinical trials and have proven very safe and are extremely well tolerated by patients. They reduce the symptoms of abdominal pain, bloating, lack of appetite and nausea associated with liver and digestive disorders. Thinking about Moringa's benefits in hepatitis (traditionally used as such in India and other countries); I believe it is very possible that its beneficial hepatoprotector effects are due precisely to the presence of these potent antioxidant and pharmacologically active caffeoylquinic acids.

SUMMARY

During normal biological processes inside our bodies, unstable molecules—free radicals—are created. They attack every cell and damage the biological structures made of lipids, proteins and genetic material.

Antioxidants produced by the body and supplied by food have to act promptly to stop the harm inflicted by free radicals at all levels.

The pollution and the stress of modern life (including poor diets) increase the oxidative stress and the production of free radicals.

Moringa contains potent antioxidants such as the carotenoids (lutein, beta-carotene, xanthins), vitamins (C, E and A), minerals (selenium) and other phytochemicals (quercetin, rutin and caffeoylquinic acids).

Complex mixtures of naturally occurring antioxidants from plants are the most effective and beneficial protectors against oxidation and aging of the tissues.

Diets including plenty of greens, vegetables, fruits and seeds have been linked with serious health benefits and a much lower incidence of various diseases.

"What we are doing to the forests of the world is but a mirror reflection of what we are doing to ourselves and to one another."

Gandhi

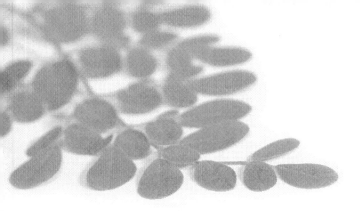

FINAL THOUGHTS
AND CONCLUSIONS

Although it is hard to say good bye to my friend, Moringa, I have to. Actually, Moringa will stay with me forever, as she remains with so many other people, as well. For the purpose of this book, though, I have to finish somewhere. I know some will read the beginning and the end first, in order to decide if they are truly interested in the whole book. In any case, closing remarks are always important - many readers will only remember those over the long run.

Before summarizing the many wonders of Moringa, I would like to expand more and explain why a plant-based diet is so important in the prevention of serious, chronic diseases, against which, we have poor weapons (read treatments). I am not going to throw too many numbers and statistics at you, I have done it already; besides, you can find the cited articles in the references if you need more details. My call is for sound thinking and, above all, inspiration from Nature, which is the greatest, most successful, oldest scientist of all. The most compassionate physician, as well!

We humans ARE part of Nature, there is no other "external" environment, we are the environment. As such, we should function according to the basic rules of Nature for proper physical and mental health. Since we were meant to eat mostly plants, as omnivorous creatures, the best way to remain functional and healthy is to continue ingesting mostly plants, especially non-cooked plants. Have you ever seen an obese wild monkey or a depressed bear (except for those in cages...)? What about hypertension, cancer or atherosclerosis in our closest omnivorous cousins? No, for as long as they have the choice, our wild relatives will choose the right food. They will eat the food that keeps their legs agile, eyes sharp, and their bodies cancer-free. The only situation in which wild animals get cancer is when they are exposed to human-created pollution. (Funny, I think, how we create the pollution that sickens us with asthma and cancer, then we struggle in so many other ways to fight these diseases, instead of addressing the cause and cleaning our internal and external environments.)

Some might argue that animals feed while humans "eat". In other words we have transformed the basic ingestion of nutrients into a social, sophisticated event; we seek the pleasure and satisfaction (taste) above all. I personally think it is the lack of basic nutrition education that leaves some ignorant or indifferent to their true organic needs. The other main reason is the total dissociation from Nature, or our own roots and who we really are. The consequences are many and sad, among these - a plethora of chronic diseases and physical weaknesses.

In the case of cancer, for instance, it is clear now that most types of cancer can be prevented or delayed by a healthy life style, especially a diet rich in vitamins and antioxidants. Healthy life style also means natural or "normal" - as normal as it used to be when we enjoyed clean food, water and air, and were forced to move a lot. Did you know that **there are thousands and thousands of scientific studies and publications about what can inhibit and how cancer can be prevented by various plants or plant-derived substances?** By contrast, there is not a single study showing that animal-based food can prevent cancers, on the contrary! Even baked foods (such as bread) and grilled meat have proven to contain cancer-promoting substances. I do not mean to scare you, but rather to draw your attention to a crucial aspect of our diet and how is it connected to our poor state of health, from poor eye sight to cancer and heart disease.

If I have to choose the single most important group of substances that are really needed but are not well represented in the Western diet, I would select the antioxidants from plants. Or, better, I would say, eat a lot of non-cooked plants! Green or colorful, canned or not, fresh better than cooked (although sometimes cooking preserves certain antioxidants), organic if possible, or whatever you can afford, just get back to your roots and eat what you were designed to eat for the best physical and mental state. You would be surprised to notice the positive changes and the energy you will draw from plants. If you are still skeptical, I say this to you; "no matter what your dietary education or habits are, if you really eat properly, when you get up from the table you should feel light, energized and clear-minded." In the long run, you should:

- rarely suffer from colds, constipation, migraines.

- have fewer wrinkles and joint pains, no need for eye glasses.

- definitely have no heartburn, high cholesterol or hypertension, to name just a few health troubles.

If you suffer from any of these, your diet is not what it is supposed to be.

I still cannot understand those who continue to eat a specific type of food no matter what clear signs of stomach distress they might get afterwards. The pill against heartburn will not stop the erosion of the gastric mucosa following a stupidly chosen meal. Even more, remember -plant-derived foods will not distress your stomach, they will protect the gastric mucosa (unless it is already ruined by previous poor eating habits). The distress most likely comes from the animal - based foods you eat.

I, for one, if science and Nature would prove that by eating stones one could prevent cancer, I would definitely stick with the stones. I have seen enough suffering...fortunately, Nature provided a much tastier alternative -the PLANTS - so I stick with them. Statistically, did you know that one in three Americans might get cancer today? These statistics look even worse for the future: in 30-50 years, one in two Americans will probably have cancer! What about in 100 years? I do not know, but what I know is that humans are not guaranteed perpetual survival. On the contrary, we are just one of many other animal species and, according to science, more than 90 % of species that have ever lived on earth have already vanished. I also know that, the further we stray from our natural eating habits, the weaker and more prone to diseases we become. Draw your own conclusions and act accordingly.

I briefly expose these serious health threats and their link to Western diet, for a better appreciation of plant derived food and - the role Moringa could play in it. You can continue to eat what you ate before, or you could ponder better alternatives. I personally trust plants to keep me healthy and energetic, the way I trust Nature to show me the path of wisdom in everything. After all, Nature has experimented on a large scale, and successfully created a myriad of opportunities and solutions for hundreds of millions of years! Among them - the Miracle Tree - Moringa. We humans have played and experimented with food for just a few thousand years or so (while junk food is much younger, of course). We started to invent and synthesize medicines less than 100 years ago...

This rather short book introduces you to *Moringa oleifera,* an unusually beneficial tree, in so many ways. My wish is that, upon reading it, you can understand her nutritional and medicinal value, and begin to appreciate Earth's amazing, still largely unknown green heritage. I have collected and put together information about Moringa's world-spread fame, extraordinary medicinal and nutritive qualities, and why her introduction into our diet could be so valuable. I mean human and animal diet. I hope to have covered the most significant data and selected the most interesting facts, although I cannot claim to have covered all, or satisfied everybody. Please keep in mind that Moringa is studied and grown in many parts of the world, within various climates and conditions; therefore, the biological data and nutritive contents can vary widely from place to place.

Besides this book, there are other valuable resources on Moringa out there, many web sites and related articles, cooking recipes, seed sources and others. Please review the "References and Resources of Information on Moringa". The book "Moringa, Nature's Medicine Cabinet" by S. Holst includes many cooking recipes using various parts of the plant.

Unfortunately, it is very difficult to find fresh Moringa on our Western markets, but one can find canned or frozen pods in gourmet stores and some Asian markets. I plan to keep growing this wonderful plant for a continuous supply in my own house, although I hope some day we will have a readily available, tasty Moringa product. Wouldn't it be wonderful to enjoy a Moringa beverage or snack daily?

Let me remind you again why this plant could be so valuable for each and every one of us, from East or West:

Moringa oleifera is extremely rich in vital nutrients, and, as a bonus, can grow very fast even in dry areas of the world, where food is scarce. Since ancient times, she was used as a medicinal plant, known to heal and ease a wide number of diseases: from various inflammations to cancer, from parasitic diseases to diabetes. In more recent times, Moringa has gained notoriety as a nutrition power plant that can feed the needy and, in fact, save lives. And eyes… from blindness due to lack of vital nutrients such as vitamin A in the diet. Moringa leaves or leaf powder can be used successfully as a complex food to nourish small children, pregnant or nursing women, and, of course, anybody else. In terms of nutrients, the leaves contain all the essential amino acids, present in harmonious combinations and significant amounts, readily bioavailable. Moringa can be, from this point of view, better than or at least as good as soy beans and soy protein.

Moringa seeds are rich in an excellent oil, very similar in quality and composition to olive oil, one of the healthiest, most studied fatty foods. The replacement of animal fats in the diet with vegetal fats such as olive or related oils has been clearly linked with beneficial health effects and reduction in cardiovascular diseases and cancers. The list of Moringa's nutrients goes on: essential minerals such as calcium, potassium, iron, and selenium, are present in Moringa, often more abundantly than in most plant sources we know of so far. Iron is much higher in Moringa than in spinach, for instance. Vitamins C, B1, B2, E, and pro-vitamin A are also present in significant quantities that make oranges or carrots pale by comparison. In addition, Moringa contains numerous phytochemicals (specific plant-derived chemicals) that act as antioxidants or antiaging substances, stimulating rejuvenation of skin and mucosa, or energizing and detoxifying the body. These beneficial substances are hormones (zeatin), others and plant pigments (flavonoids) such as rutin and quercetin, to name just a few. All these naturally occurring nutrients and medicines of Moringa are known to be best absorbed and active in the body if derived from natural sources (such as plants), and are present in complex combinations. Many of these beneficial substances act synergistically, enhancing each other's properties.

Not less exciting are Moringa's medicinal properties, as described in the chapter dedicated to the medicinal uses of this plant around the world. What is more interesting is that science continues to validate the ancient traditional therapeutic uses of Moringa. Recently, novel derivatives of thiocarbamates and nitriles which stimulate insulin release in animals have been found in Moringa. These compounds and their action explain the anti-diabetic properties of the Miracle Tree. The list with valuable, recent medicinal discoveries related to Moringa goes on and on. One would need hundreds of pages to mention all the discoveries and describe their content.

Now that you understand better the value of this plant to us, you might consider as justified all those suggestive, affectionate names people gave Moringa: "Miracle Tree," "Mother's Best Friend," and "Never Die." I could not think of a better name…

After so much talk about food, you must be hungry...
Enjoy your meal!

I will enjoy my Moringa.

REFERENCES AND RESOURCES OF INFORMATION ON MORINGA

Introducing Moringa
Moringa in the News

The Miracle Tree. *Moringa oleifera:* Natural Nutrition for the Tropics, Lowell J. Fuglie, regional representative, Church World Service; Dakar, Senegal; Moringa Tree Project, Church World Service, 1999.

Moringa Tree Could Reduce Malnutrition in Africa United Methodist News Service, (UMNS), April 24, 2000.

New crops: Solutions for global problems -Vietmeyer, N. pp. 2-8; J. Janick (ed.), Progress in new crops. ASHS Press, Alexandria, Virginia, 1996.

Nutritive Value of Indian Foods, Gopalan et al; Hyderabad, India, National Institute of Nutrition, Indian Council of Medical Research, 1989.

Moringa oleifera: A Tree and a Litany of Potential, Folkard, Geoff, Sutherland, John, Agroforestry Today, Vol. 8, No. 3, July-September 1996, pp. 5-8.

Moringa, Nature's Medicine Cabinet, Sanford Holst, Sierra Sunrise Publishing, 2000.

Miracle tree has spread its roots, Calovich, Annie; The Wichita Eagle, May 31, 2000, p. A1.

Gnarly tree can cure the ill, purify water and feed the hungry, A Common Tree with Rare Power, Fritz, Mark, Los Angeles Times, March 27, 2000, pp. A1, A14.

Moringa: a miracle tree for developing countries?, Bazeley, B.W. , "The Rotarian", February 1999, p. 6.

The Drumstick Tree: A Natural Multi-Vitamin -Moringa tree cheap solution to malnutrition in Africa, Sreenivasan, Jyotsna , The Environmental Magazine, May, 2000.

Moringa oleifera as a natural coagulant, Sutherland, J.P., Folkard, G.K., Mtawali, M.A., Grant, W.D.; Pickford, et al. eds., Affordable Water Supply & Sanitation: Proceedings of the 20th WEDC Conference, Colombo, Sri Lanka, pp. 22-6, August 1994.

Moringa oleifera – an underutilized tree with amazing versatility, Becker, K.

Drumstic *(Moringa oleifera):* A multipurpose Indian vegetable, Ramachandran, C., Peter, K.V. and Gopalakrishan, P. K.; Economic Botany, 34 (3), pp. 276-83, 1980.

The potential of *Moringa oleifera* for agricultural and industrial uses, Foidl, N., Makkar, H.P.S. and Becker. K.; Communication at "Development potential for Moringa products ", Dar es Salaam, Tanzania, Octo-ber-November, 2001.

The Moringa Tree, Price, M. L., ECHO Technical note, 2000.

Moringa oleifera - an underutilised tree with amazing versatility, Becker, K., Workgroup Multifunctional Plants - Food, Feed, Industrial Products, Indonesia, 2003.

And numerous web sites dedicated to *Moringa oleifera*.

Moringa, the Medicinal Plant

Moringa, Nature's Medicine Cabinet, Sanford Holst, Sierra Sunrise Publishing, 2000.

Hypotensive constituents from the pods of Moringa oleifera, Faizi, S., et al., Planta Med., April, Vol. 64, p. 225, 1998.

Studies on the antiulcer activity of *Moringa oleifera* leaf extract on gastric ulcer models in rats, Pal, S.K., Mukherjee, P.K. and Saha, B.P., Phytotherapy Research, Vol. 9, pp. 463-65, 1995.

The antibiotic principle of seeds of *Moringa oleifera*. and *Moringa stenopetala,* Eilert, U., et al., Planta Res., Vol.42, pp. 55-61, 1981.

Studies on the anti-inflammatory and wound healing properties of *Moringa oleifera* and *Aegle marmelos,* Udupa, S.L. et al., Fitoterapia, 65 (2), pp.119-23, 1994.

Plants used against cancer. A survey, Hartwell J.L., Lloydia, pp. 30-40,1967-1971.

Hypotensive constituents from the pods of *Moringa oleifera,* Faizi, S., et al., Planta Med., April, 64 (3), pp. 225-28, 1998.

Isolation and structure elucidation of new nitrile and mustard oil glycosides from *Moringa oleifera* and their effect on blood pressure, Faizi, S., et al., Journal of Natural Products, 57 (9), pp. 1256-261, 1994.

Modulatory potency of drumstick lectin on the host defense system, Jayavardhanan, K.K., et al., J. Exp. Clin. Cancer Res., 13 (3), pp. 205-09, 1994.

The horseradish tree, *Moringa pterygosperma* (Moringaceae) - A boon to arid lands? Morton, J. F., Economic Botany, 45 (3), pp. 318-33, 1991.

Niaziminin, a thiocarbamate from the leaves of *Moringa oleifera,* holds a strict structural requirement for inhibition of tumor-promoter-induced Epstein-Barr virus activation., Murakami, A., et al., Planta Med., May; 64 (4), pp. 319-23, 1998.

Antioxidant Action of *Moringa oleifera Lam* (Drumstick) Against Antitubercular Drugs Induced Lipid Peroxidation in Rats, N. Ashok Kumar, Journal of Medicinal Food, October, Vol. 6, No. 3, pp. 255-59, 2003.

Pharmacological studies of thiocarbamate glycosides isolated from *Moringa oleifera* Jansakul, Chaweewan, et al., J. Sci. Soc. Thailand, 1997, 23, pp. 335-46, 1997.

Pharmacological investigations on aqueous extract of *Moringa pterygosperma,* Limaye, D.A., et al., Phytotherapy Research, 8, 37, 1995.

Hypocholesterolemic effects of crude extract of leaf of *Moringa oleifera Lam* in high-fat diet fed wistar rats. Nwobodo, Ghasi S., et al., J. Ethnopharmacol., January; 69 (1), pp. 21-25, 2000.

An antitumor promoter from *Moringa oleifera Lam.,* Guevara, A.P., et al., Mutat Res., April 6; 440 (2), pp. 181-88, 1999.

Moringa, the Nutritive Plant

Biochemistry, Berg, Jeremy M., Stryer, Lubert, Tymoczko, John L., Published Freeman, W.H., ISBN 0716730510, 2002.

Advanced Nutrition and Human Metabolism, Groff, J.L., Gropper, S.S., Hunt, S.M., West Publishing Company, New York, 1995.

Nutritional Value of Drumstick Leaves, The Trees For Life Organization.

Moringa, a highly nutritious vegetable tree, Ram, J., Tropical Rural and Island/Atoll Development Experimental Station (TRIADES), Technical Bulletin No. 2 , 1994.

Drumstick *(Moringa oleifera):* A multipurpose Indian Vegetable. Ramachandran, C., et al., Economic Botany, 34 (3) pp. 276-83, 1980.

Nutritional value of Moringa, Verma, S.C., et al., Current Sci. 45 (21) pp. 769-70, 1976.

The horseradish tree, *Moringa pterygosperma* (Moringaceae) -A boon to arid lands? Morton, J.F., Economic Botany, 45 (3), pp. 318-33, 1991.

Nutrients and anti-quality factors in different morphological parts of the *Moringa oleifera* tree, Makkar, H.

P.S., and Becker, K., Journal of Agricultural Sciences (Cambridge), 128, pp.311-22, 1997.

Moringa, Nature's Medicine Cabinet, Sanford Holst, Sierra Sunrise Publishing, 2000.

Nutritional value and antinutritional components of whole and ethanol extracted *Moringa oleifera* leaves, H. P. S. Makkar and K. Becker, Animal Feed Science and Technology, Vol. 63, Issues 1-4, December, pp. 211-228, 1996.

The potential of *Moringa oleifera* for agricultural and industrial uses, Foidl, N., Makkar, H.P.S. and Becker, K.; Communication at "Development potential for Moringa products ", Dar es Salaam, Tanzania, Octo-ber-November, 2001.

The Miracle Tree. *Moringa oleifera:* Natural Nutrition for the Tropics. Fuglie, Lowell J., regional representative, Church World Service, Dakar, Senegal, Moringa Tree Project, Church World Service, 1999.

Moringa olifeira - an underutilised tree with amazing versatility, Becker, K., Workgroup Multifunctional Plants - Food, Feed, Industrial Products, Indonesia, 2003.

Combating micronutrient deficiencies: problems and perspectives., Alnwick, D.J., Proc. Nutr. Soc. 57, pp. 137-47, 1998.

Nutrition: the global challenge. FAO-WHO., International Conference of Nutrition, 5-11, Rome, December 1992.

Nutritional evaluation of protein foods, Edited by Pellett, Peter L. and Young, Vernon R. , The United Nations University, 1980.

Recommended Dietary Allowances, Food and Nutrition Board, National Research Council, 10th ed., Washington, DC: National Academy Press, 1989.

Diet and Health. Implications for Reducing Chronic Disease, Committee on Diet and Health, Food and Nutrition Board: Washington, DC: National Academy Press, 1989.

Bioavailability: A factor in protein quality, Kies, C., J. Agric. Food Chem.; 29: pp. 435-40, 1981.

Position of The American Dietetic Association: Vegetarian diets. J. Am. Diet Assoc., 97, pp. 1317321, 1997.

Dietary reference intakes for energy, carbohydrate, fiber, fat, fatty acids, cholesterol, protein, and amino acids, Institute of Medicine, Washington, DC, National Academies Press, 2002.

Dietary protein increases urinary calcium, Kerstetter, JE, Allen, LH., J. Nutr.; 120: pp. 134-36, 1990.

Proteins, Peptides and Amino Acids Source Book, White, John S., White, Dorothy C., Humana Press, 2002.

Plant proteins in relation to human protein and amino acid nutrition. Young, V.R., Pellett, P.L. Am. J. Clin. Nutr; 59 (suppl), pp. 1203S-212S, 1994.

The effect of milk supplements on calcium metabolism, bone metabolism and calcium balance, Recker, R.R., Heaney, R.P., American Journal of Clinical Nutrition, Vol. 41, pp. 254-63, 1985.

Advanced Nutrition and Human Metabolism, Groff, J.L., Gropper, S.S., Hunt, S.M., West Publishing Company, New York, 1995.

Calcium Factor: The Scientific Secret of Health & Youth, Barefoor, Robert R. and Reich, Carl J. , Triad Marketing, 2002.

An association between osteoporosis and premenstrual symptoms and postmenopausal symptoms, Lee, S.J., Kanis, J.A., Bone and Mineral; 24, pp. 127-34, 1994.

The Miracle of Magnesium, Dean, Carolyn , Random House, USA, Inc., 2003.

Iron Deficiency Anemia: Recommended Guidelines for the Prevention, Detection, and Management Among U.S. Children and Women of Childbearing Age, Woteki, Robert Earl and Catherine E. Editors, Institute of Medicine, 1993.

Battling Iron Deficiency Anaemia, World Health Organization, Geneva, Switzerland, 2000.

Dietary fat and cancer, Kushi, L., Giovannucci, E. Am. J. Med., 113 Suppl. 9B: pp. 63S-70S, 2002.

Diet, lifestyle, and the risk of type 2 diabetes mellitus in women, Hu F.B., et al., N. Engl. J. Med., 345, pp. 790-97, 2001.

Types of dietary fat and risk of coronary heart disease: a critical review, Hu F.B., et al., J. Am. Coll. Nutr., 20, pp. 5-19, 2001.

Flax oil as a true aid against arthritis, heart infarction, cancer and other diseases, Budwig, J., Apple Publishing, 1982.

Intake of trans fatty acids and risk of coronary heart disease among women , Willett, W.C., et al., Lancet, 341, pp. 581-85, 1996.

Types of dietary fat and breast cancer: a pooled analysis of cohort studies, Smith-Warner, et al., Int. J. Cancer; 92, pp. 767-74, 2001.

Diet and cancer-an overview, Willett, W.C, MacMahon, B., N. Engl. J. Med.; 310, pp. 633-38, 1984 and (two parts). N. Engl. J. Med., 310, pp. 697703, 1984.

Characterization of *Moringa oleifera* variety Mbololo seed oil of Kenya, Tsaknis J. et al., J. Agric Food Chem., November, 47 (11) pp. 4495-499, 1999.

Olive Oil Cookery: The Mediterranean Diet, Abbas, Maher A., Farquhar, John W., Book Publishing Company (TN), 1995.

The Diet and 15-Year Death Rate in the Seven Countries, Keys, A., et al., H.; Study. Am. J. Epidemiol. 124, pp. 903-15, 1986.

Olive Oil and the Mediterranean Diet: Implications for Health in Europe, Assmann, G., et al., Br. J. Nurs., 6, pp. 675-77, 1997.

Mediterranean Dietary Pattern in a Randomized Trial: Prolonged Survival and Possible Reduced Cancer Rate, de Lorgeril, M., et al., Arch. Intern. Med., 158, pp. 1181-187, 1998.

Olive Oil and Reduced Need for Antihypertensive Medications, Ferrara, L., et al., Arch. Intern. Med., 160, pp. 837-42, 2000.

Dietary Fat, Olive Oil Intake and Breast Cancer Risk, Martin-Moreno, J. M., et al., Int. J. Cancer, 58, pp. 774-80, 1994.

Protective Effects Upon Experimental Inflammation Models of a Polyphenol-Supplemented Virgin Olive Oil Diet, Martinez-Dominguez, E., de la, P. R., Ruiz-Gutierrez, V., Inflamm. Res., 50, pp. 102-06, 2001.

Antiatherogenic Components of Olive Oil., Visioli, F., Galli, C., Curr. Atheroscler. Rep. 3, pp. 64-67, 2001.

Evidence-Based Approach to Vitamins and Minerals: Health Implications and Intake Recommendations, Higdon, Jane, Thieme Medical Pub., 2003.

Encyclopedia of Vitamins, Minerals and Supplements, Navarra, Tova, Publisher: Facts on File, Inc., 1996.

The Vitamin Sourcebook, Reinhard, Tonia, Publisher: McGraw-Hill Companies, 1998.

Cancer and Vitamin C, Cameron E., and Linus P., Camino Books, Philadelphia, 1993.

The neural activity of thiamine: facts and hypotheses, Parkhomenko, I.M., et al. , 68(2): pp. 3-14, 1996.

Food chemistry, Fennema, O.R., Second edition, Dekker, M., New York, 1985.

Toxic effects of water-soluble vitamins, Alhadeff, L., et al., Nutr Rev. 42, pp. 33-40, 1984.

Thiamin and the brain, Haas, RH., Ann. Rev. Nutr., 8: pp. 483-515, 1988.

Degradation of thiamine and riboflavin during extrusion processing. , Beetner, G.T., et al., A research note., J. Food Sci.; 39: pp. 207-08, 1974.

Plasma levels of lipophilic antioxidants in very old patients with type 2 diabetes, Polidori, M.C., et al., Diabetes Metab Res. Rev., 16, pp. 15-9, 2000.

Beta-carotene supplementation and incidence of cancer and cardiovascular disease: the Women's Health Study, Lee, I.M., et al., J. Natl. Cancer Inst. 91, pp. 2102-106, 1999.

Lack of effect of long-term supplementation with beta carotene on the incidence of malignant neoplasms and cardiovascular disease, Hennekens, C.H., et al., N. Engl. J. Med., 334: pp. 1145-149, 1996.

Recommended dietary intakes (RDI) of vitamin A in humans, Olson, J.A., Am. J. Clin. Nutr., Vol. 45, pp. 704-16, 1987.

Bioavailability of a natural isomer mixture compared with synthetic all-trans beta-carotene in human serum, Ben-Amotz, A., Levy, Y., Am. J. Clin. Nutr., 63, pp. 729-34, 1996.

Nutrition and cancer: A review of the evidence for an anti-cancer diet, Donaldson, Michael S., Nutr. J., October 20;3 (1) : p. 19, 2004.

Effect of dietary phytochemicals on cancer development, Waladkhani, A.R., Clemens, M.R., Int. J. Mol. Med., April;1 (4) : pp. 747-53, 1998.

The role of phytotherapy in treating lower urinary tract symptoms and benign prostatic hyperplasia., Dreikorn, K., World J. Urol., April, 19 (6): pp. 426-35, 2002.

The beneficial effects of plant sterols on serum cholesterol., Wong, N.C., Can. J. Cardiol. June, 17 (6), pp. 715-21, 2001.

Control of differentiation and apoptosis of human myeloid leukemia cells by cytokinins and cytokinin nucleosides, plant redifferentiation-inducing hormones. Ishii, Y., Honma, Y., et al., Cell Growth Differ., January,13 (1), pp. 19-26, 2002.

Differentiation of human myeloid leukemia cells by plant redifferentiation-inducing hormones, Honma, Y., Ishii, Y., Leuk Lymphoma., September; 43(9), pp.1729-735, 2002.

Phytohormones and Related Compounds - A Comprehensive Treatise", Elsevier. Edited by Letham, D.S., Goodwin, P.B. and Higgins, T.J.V., 1978.

Kinetin delays the onset of aging characteristics in human fibroblasts. Rattan, S.I., Clark, B.F., Biochem. biophys. Res. Commun., 201, pp. 665-72, 1994.

The cellular and molecular biology of skin aging., West M.I.D., Arch. Dermatol., 130: pp. 87-95, 1994.

Cell aging., Hayflick, L., In Eisdorfer C (ed), Annual Review of Gerontology and Geriatrics, Vol. 1, Springer Publishing, New York, pp. 26-67, 1980.

Kinetin inhibits protein oxidation and glycoxidation in vitro., Verbeke, P., et al., Biochem. Biophys. Res. Commun., October 5; 276 (3), pp. 1265-270, 2000.

Plant growth hormone kinetin delays aging, prolongs the lifespan and slows down development of the fruitfly *Zaprionus Paravittiger*, Sharma, S.P., Kaur, P., Rattan, S.I., Biochem. Biophys. Res. Commun., November 22, 216 (3), pp. 1067-71, 1995.

Inhibitory mechanisms of kinetin, a plant growth-pro-moting hormone, in platelet aggregation, Sheu, J.R., Hsiao, G., et al., Platelets, May, 14 (3): pp. 189-96., 2003.

Cosmeceuticals, Kligman, D., Dermatol. Clin., October, 18 (4), pp. 609-15, 2000.

Influence of kinetin (6-furfurylo-amino-purine) on human fibroblasts in the cell culture, Kowalska, E., Folia. Morphol. (Warsz), 51 (2), pp. 109-18, 1992.

Inhibitory effect of zeatin, isolated from *Fiatoua villosa,* on acetylcholinesterase activity from PC12 cells., Heo, H.J., Hong, S.C., et al., Mol. Cells., February, 28, 13 (1), pp. 113-17, 2002.

Zeatin, a factor inducing cell division isolated from Zea mays. Letham, D.S., Life Sci. 8, pp. 569-73, 1963.

The structure of zeatin, a factor inducing cell division, Letham, D. S et al., Proc. Chem. Soc. (Lond.), pp. 23031, 1964.

A Cancer Therapy - Results of Fifty Cases and The Cure of Advanced Cancer by Diet Therapy - A Summary of 30 Years of Clinical Experimentation, Gerson, M.D., Max Gerson Institute, Binita, California, 1990.

Antioxidant properties of various solvent extracts of total phenolic constituents from three different agroclimatic origins of drumstick tree *(Moringa oleifera Lam.)* leaves, Siddhuraju, P., Becker, K., J. Agric. Food. Chem., April, 9;51 (8), pp. 2144-155, 2003.

Importance Of Good Nutrition, Herbs And Phytochemicals: For Your Health, Good Looks, Ambau, Getty T., Falcon Press International.

Free Radicals in Medicine, Olinescu, Radu, Nova Science Pub., Inc., June 2000.

Super Anti-Oxidants: Why They Will Change the Face of Healthcare in the 21st Century, Balch, James F., Natl. Book Network, 1999.

Antioxidant Status, Diet, Nutrition, and Health, Papas, Andreas M., CRC Press, 1998.

Profiling glucosinolates and phenolics in vegetative and reproductive tissues of the multi-purpose trees *Moringa oleifera L.* (horseradish tree) and *Moringa stenopetala,* Bennett, R.N., et al., J. Agric. Food. Chem., June 4, 51 (12), pp. 3546-553, 2003.

Chlorogenic acid and caffeic acid are absorbed in humans, Olthof, M.R., Hollman, P.C., Katan, M.B., J. Nutr., January, 131 (1), pp. 66-71, 2001.

Quercetin protects cutaneous tissue-associated cell types including sensory neurons from oxidative stress induced by glutathione depletion: cooperative effects of ascorbic acid. Skaper, S.D., Fabris, M., et al., Free Radic. Biol. Med., 22 (4), pp. 669-78, 1997.

An ideal ocular nutritional supplement? Bartlett, H., Eperjesi, F., Ophthalmic Physiol. Opt. July, 24 (4), pp. 339-49, 2004.

The science behind lutein, Alves-Rodrigues, A., Shao, A., Toxicol Lett., April 15, 150 (1), pp. 57-83, 2004.

Antimutagens, anticarcinogens, and effective worldwide cancer prevention, Weisburger, J.H., J. Environ. Pathol. Toxicol. Oncol., 18 (2), pp. 85-93, 1999.

Fruits and vegetables in the prevention of cellular oxidative damage. Prior, R.L., Am. J. Clin. Nutr., September, 78, (3 Suppl), pp. 570S-78S. Review, 2003.

Insulin Secretagogues from *Moringa oleifera* with Cyclooxygenase Enzyme and Lipid Peroxidation Inhibitory Activities, Jayaraj, A. Francis, Bolleddula Jayaprakasam, et al., Helvetica Chimica. Acta., Vol. 87, 2, pp. 317-26, February, 2004.

Cancer Facts and Figures 2004, Thun, MD, Michael J., epidemiology and surveillance research, American Cancer Society, Atlanta, 2004.

The High Stakes of Cancer Prevention, Epstein, Samuel, Gross, Liza, Tikkun Magazine, November/ December 2000.

Index

D

Dementia 112, 113
Depression 41, 42, 51, 67, 70
Detoxification 40, 77, 97
Detoxify 54, 55
Diabetes 69, 90, 141, 154, 157

E

EFA's/Essential Fatty Acids 65, 70, 71
Elderly 127, 130

F

FAO 33, 36, 44, 152
Fats
  Saturated Fats 49, 65, 66, 68, 69
  Unsaturated Fats 67
Fat-Soluble 74, 90, 125, 127
Fatty Acids 30, 53, 65, 70, 71, 123, 152, 154
Fiber 29, 152
Flavonoids 15, 128, 129, 143
Food and Agricultural Organization 33
Free Radicals 60, 77, 89, 90, 106, 121, 122, 124, 126, 132
Fruit 86

G

Genetically Modified (GM) 34, 44
Glucose 5, 43, 53, 55, 69
Glutathione 55, 162
Glycine 55
Glycosides 18, 148, 149

H

Hair 40, 55, 104, 111
Heart Disease 20, 49, 51, 55, 67, 68, 70, 71, 77, 78, 87, 90,

Lutein 30, 120, 125, 126, 127, 132, 162
Lysine 36, 39

—————— **M** ——————

Magnesium xi, 50, 51, 153
Malnutrition 9, 10, 146
Manganese xi, 61
Mediterranean 68, 155
Men 51, 128
Metabolism 15, 40, 43, 50, 53, 62, 79, 82, 83, 108, 112, 153
Methionine 33, 36, 39, 40, 55
Migraine 42
Milk xv, 11, 21, 28, 29, 33, 34, 48, 49, 87, 153
Muscles 38, 43, 50, 58, 60, 79

—————— **N** ——————

Nausea 51, 131
Nerves 79, 83
Neuronal 112, 113, 116
Niacin 42
Niaziminin 17, 149
Nicotinic Acid 83
Nitriles 143
Nutrition 31, 145, 150, 151, 152, 153, 158, 161
Nutritional Value 24

—————— **O** ——————

Obesity 24, 41
Oleic Acid 65
Optima of Africa, Ltd. 24
Osteoarthritis 40, 41
Osteoporosis 47